Australian Edition

The HUNGER HERO DIET: How to Lose Weight and Break the Depression Cycle

– Without Exercise, Drugs, or Surgery

Kathryn M. James

Copyright © 2022 by Kathryn M James

All Rights Reserved.
No part of this book may be used or reproduced by any means, graphic, electronic, or mechanical, including photocopying, recording, taping, or by any information storage retrieval system without the written permission of the copyright owner, except in the case of brief quotations embodied in critical articles and reviews.

The Working Alliance , Gold Coast, Australia
ISBN 978-0-6455255-1-9
Australian Edition

kmjameswriter.com

The Australian Edition contains product information specific to the supermarket shopping experience in Australasia.

Disclaimer

Neither the author nor the publisher can be held liable to any person or entity with respect to any loss or damage caused, or alleged to be caused, directly or indirectly, by the information contained in this work or associated media. As any scientist will affirm, results may vary, so no guarantee is given or implied with regard to information supplied. It is general information only.

It is not the intent of the author to diagnose or prescribe. The intent is only to offer health information to help you cooperate with your medical professionals in your mutual quest for health. In the event you use this information without their approval, you are prescribing for yourself, which is your right, but the publisher and author assume no responsibility. While every precaution has been taken to ensure the information presented herein is accurate, there are many factors beyond the control of the author.

Before starting any diet, you should speak to your doctor. Do not rely on information in this book as an alternative to medical advice. If you have any specific questions about any medical matter, consult your medical practitioner.

All trademarks or brand names mentioned by the author, in this book or elsewhere, remain unreservedly the property of their respective owners, and no claim is made to them, and no endorsement by them is implied or claimed.

Table of Contents

INTRODUCTION...7

Chapter 1: Promises, promises...13

Chapter 2: Under the knife...37

Chapter 3: Reality check..46

Chapter 4: Diet is not a dirty word..57

Chapter 5: Superfoods – fact or fiction?..............................72

Chapter 6: Who gets it right?..89

Chapter 7: How did you get so fat?...................................109

Chapter 8: How much is enough?......................................127

Chapter 9: Are you ready for change?..............................139

Chapter 10: Strive to become your best self....................149

Chapter 11: Self-care for mind and body.........................164

Chapter 12: Secrets of success..171

    RULE 1: Tick tock, watch the clock.............................173

    RULE 2: Repeat, repeat, repeat.....................................176

    RULE 3: Be mindful – stay focused..............................178

    RULE 4: Size does matter...182

    RULE 5: Keep track with your DIET DIARY............185

    RULE 6: Follow the Rules..189

Chapter 13: Hunger Hero MENU PLAN..........................192

    Morning fast and cleanse...194

    Lunch: 11.30am-12 noon..196

    Afternoon snack: 2.30pm...198

Dinner: 5.30-6pm...200

Evening snack: 7-7.30pm..202

Chapter 14: The HUNGER HEROES................................203

Chapter 15: Hunger Hero RECIPES..................................216

    How to fold RICE PAPERS..217

    LUNCH RECIPES...220

        Recipe: Tinned TUNA rice paper rolls...................221

        Recipe: PRAWN rice paper rolls.............................223

    LUNCH VARIATIONS...226

        Recipe: Poached EGGS & braised veg....................230

        Recipe: Mediterranean tomato salad......................232

    AFTERNOON SNACKS...233

    DINNER RECIPES..237

        Recipe: Pan-seared TUNA STEAK........................238

        Recipe: Pan-fried thin WHITE FISH.......................240

        Recipe: Crispy skin SALMON fillet........................242

    DINNER VARIATIONS...244

        Recipe: Thick WHITE FISH, braised veg...............247

        Recipe: Pan-fried PORK scotch fillet......................249

        Recipe: Stuffed MUSHROOM CAPS....................251

        Recipe: Grilled VEGETABLES................................254

    RICE NOODLE DISHES..258

        Dry bowl, wet bowl, or soup broth........................262

        Recipe: The Traveller, TUNA noodle salad........... 263

Recipe: TUNA steak & tomato noodle salad........ 264

Recipe: TUNA steak & veg noodle bowl................265

Recipe: PORK & avocado salad noodle bowl....... 267

Recipe: PRAWN & braised veg noodle bowl........268

Recipe: PRAWN & Asian greens noodle broth.... 269

EVENING SNACKS..271

Recipe: Easy AVOCADO dip.................................. 274

Chapter 16: Let's go shopping.. 275

Chapter 17: Life after dieting.. 295

References... 300

About the author...314

INTRODUCTION

From desperation to inspiration

December 2017: "The pain is killing me. Nobody will help me. Nobody cares. Nothing works. I'm sick of being depressed all the time. My weight is out of control. There are parts of my body I can't even reach. I fucking hate my life. I can't live like this."

That was me, not that long ago, writhing in pain, a prisoner of my own four walls, unable to walk or care for myself, feeling utterly helpless and hopeless.

I was alone, it was Christmas Day and the future looked bleak. I had reached the time of life that had taken my father and sister, and despite having lived a very different life to them, it seemed I could not escape my genetic destiny. I didn't have long to live, or so I thought. I could feel myself sinking deeper and deeper into the all-too-familiar black abyss of a major depressive episode, but this time it was worse. I wasn't fighting it. I had accepted my fate. I had finally given up.

But the only way is up, right? Well yeah, that's what keeps us going each day. When things get tough, we always find a way out of it. That's what it means to be a survivor – you find a way to survive. But not this time. I'd tried and failed. I couldn't take any more. Too much trauma. Too much pain. My mind just switched off. I slept and slept, then slept some more. I lost all concept of time and place. That final week of December 2017 was lost forever in a lonely fog of nothingness and despair.

Does any of this sound familiar? Has chronic pain turned your life into a nightmare? Have you stopped enjoying life, limited by fear or isolation? Do you struggle with depression, anxiety, panic attacks, post-traumatic stress, or all the above? Do you feel a deep overwhelming sense of sadness and disappointment? Are you losing control of your mind and body? Is life just too hard? I hope you never reach this point, but if you have, I hear you. And I want to share something miraculous with you.

When I finally emerged from that black hole of despair, something amazing had happened. Not only had my mood improved, but I had lost 2.8 kilograms in less than a week! I was shocked and stunned, but also excited. I thought long and hard about what I had been doing that week, and decided to keep doing it to see what would happen.

Finding hope

After that first week of losing weight, I felt energised. I wanted to understand why this was happening when everything else had failed. This started me on a hunt for answers, to find evidence of medical research to explain what was going on. I wanted to create a diet that helped control my appetite so I could lose weight, but was that even possible?

Could I create a sustainable, long-term eating plan that fulfilled all the desired elements of sweet, sour, salty, umami, bitter, crunchy, smooth, oily and fried? Could I use everyday supermarket ingredients that were easily accessible, quick to prepare, and full of nutritional goodness? Could I find something to act as an appetite suppressant between meals? Could I replace the bread that I loved so much, with something equally satisfying? Could I create a new way of eating that would solve my issues around portion control, retrain my new behaviours, and satisfy my appetite at mealtimes? YES, YES, YES, YES, YES!

That was January 2018, and by the end of February I knew I had discovered something extraordinary. After losing 10kg in only 50 days, I became aware of significant improvements in my mobility and my mental health. My arthritic pain became manageable without medication, the painful swelling around my knees and ankles had gone, and the crippling bursts of abdominal pain had eased. According to obesity research, systemic inflammation is a major factor, but in my opinion, the level of improvement far outweighed what one could expect from simply losing 10kg. While even a small weight loss will have noticeable health benefits, I believe that my chronic pain improved to such a staggering degree due to a combination of removing certain foods from my diet and replacing them with others.

By August I had lost a whopping 35kg (77 pound or 5.5 stone). I had consistently lost over a kilo a week, **without exercise**. I had literally saved my own life. Don't get me wrong; I am not lazy; I've always loved being physically active; but I was injured and in a lot of pain, so every attempt at exercise just made things worse. But for the first time in 12 years, I was walking without a stick. I no longer felt vulnerable or too afraid to leave home. I was getting my life back. I felt such an amazing sense of achievement, not just physically, but mentally as well.

Breaking the cycle of depression

But by far the most exciting and completely unexpected outcome of this new eating plan was the positive effect on my mental health. Yes of course my mood improved once I started losing weight; I felt less pain, had improved mobility, and I felt better about myself. But I soon began to realise that my regular episodic bouts of depressive malaise had shrunk from a debilitating 10 days every few weeks (when I couldn't think straight or function), to a single day when I simply felt not-quite-right. That in itself was nothing short of miraculous.

For years I used physical exercise as an antidote to my emotional problems, but that was taken away from me 14 years ago when old injuries and arthritis made every movement a painful experience. So, can you imagine what it feels like to be suddenly free?

The depression is still there, always threatening to take over again, but it remains under control as long as I keep following this eating plan – and that is my major motivator and my prize. The latest neurobiology research suggests the answer might lie in the gut microbiota, and we'll talk more about those theories throughout the book.

Sharing is caring

I know the reality of physical injury and emotional trauma, and how they feed each other to make things worse.

I know how negative experiences can trigger changes in health and physical appearance.

I know how easy it is to develop 'disordered' ways of eating – by severely restricting the types of foods we eat, or by eating too much.

I know how life can become a string of disappointments, and how it can sometimes seem all too hard.

Going public with such a personal story fills me with trepidation. I don't know how it will be received, but I hope it strikes a chord in those who might benefit. I know that by telling my story and showing my vulnerability, I risk becoming a target for ridicule and criticism. There are those who think 'fat-shaming' on social media is a team sport, but I feel compelled to speak up. I wish somebody had written this book for me years ago, before I hit rock bottom and lost hope, but maybe this book can save someone else from all that unnecessary pain and suffering.

Knowledge is power

"Give a hungry person a fish, and they'll eat for a day. Teach them to fish, and they'll have the skills to feed themselves for a lifetime". It's a rough interpretation of an ancient Chinese proverb, but it holds true even today. Knowledge is power.

My intention with this book is to provide just enough information for you to feel confident about your food choices into the future, with a few simple strategies to improve your behaviours and help you stay on track.

We share the latest scientific evidence, from peer-reviewed articles published in reputable medical research journals. Many are 'systematic reviews' that typically collate results from at least 100 original research studies on any given topic. They are the most reliable source.

While this is a resource for anyone struggling with obesity, I do tend to focus more on the needs of older women. I make no excuses for that, because I know what it feels like to be an older woman struggling with obesity and depression. But this diet plan can help anyone who has a lot of weight to lose, men and women, young or old.

Every chapter is intended to carry you forward on a journey of self-discovery, one page at a time, uncovering the mysteries of our bodies and minds.

The secret to good mental and physical health is finding BALANCE in our lives. It sounds so simple, but few of us manage the basics: a good night's sleep, some daily physical activity, quality time with friends and family, and the right kind of nutrition for our stage of life. **The Hunger Hero Diet** will show you the way. It is never too late to change.

Join me as we delve into the **Science of Food, Mood and Weight Loss**, and uncover the secrets of the **Hunger Hero Diet**. Knowledge is power! You can do this.

Chapter 1: Promises, promises

Ever wondered why diets never seem to work? Have you ever suspected you were being setup for failure? Well, the answer might shock and disappoint, but this is the inconvenient truth underpinning the diet industry. If you lose weight and keep it off, they stop making money. They expect you to fail. They want you to keep coming back to them, willing to try the next gimmick. To see if you agree, join me for a stroll down memory lane.

Weight Watchers started way back in the 1960s. This international community-based weight loss organisation was both effective and innovative, providing lifestyle education, healthy recipes, peer support and accountability, with the core message of preparing fresh food and eating three meals a day. They held members accountable at supervised weekly weigh-ins, using a 'bottom up' approach which allowed members to influence how the program evolved.

By 1978, they had become a recognisable and trusted brand, and food manufacturing giant, Heinz, stepped in for a piece of the action. They developed a line of processed freezer meals with Weight Watchers branding – becoming one of the first commercial food manufacturing companies to realise the potential of this market. The meals were single-serve and calorie-controlled, a novel idea and way ahead of its time. The microwave oven was the newest gadget in home kitchens, so it made a lot of sense.

In the 1970s, we challenged traditional female stereotypes as more women worked outside the home and gained more independence. We saw the rise of women's magazines and their shift from the traditional knitting, baking and homemaking of post-war 'Stepford wives', to a new focus on single women with interests in fashion, makeup, romance, and sexual attraction. Every month, these influential magazines flashed glamourous photos in exotic locations, of impossibly tall and lanky models draped in the most exquisite clothing, accompanied by elegant and sophisticated men. It was like living in a James Bond movie.

Our favourite magazines offered glimpses of what life could be like if we could only LOSE WEIGHT, and then exploited our naivety with promises of a new miracle diet in almost every issue. With an embarrassing eagerness, we rushed forward and gobbled up everything they fed us. We religiously stuck to the so-called Israeli Army Diet for 10 days, eating nothing but apples, chicken and salad. We believed claims about the Grapefruit Diet, which elevated the humble grapefruit to superfood status.

Diets sold magazines! And it didn't take long for American diet books to appear on the shelves beside the women's magazines. In 1979, the Pritikin Diet was an early adopter of a low-fat approach to weight loss that would have wide-ranging consequences for decades to come. Cholesterol was the first casualty in this war on fat. The humble egg became a no-go zone, so people turned to breakfast cereal, making Mr Kellogg very happy.

It was around this time that manufacturers starting tinkering with dairy products too, but while they were taking out the natural animal fats, they were adding lots of sugars and artificial additives. We turned away from natural food and embraced the artificial, thinking it was a healthy option. We believed the advertising. This was the trend in America, the land of manufacturing, and we quickly followed in their footsteps.

The 1980s saw the emergence of self-help books and the 'health guru'. It was such a hugely influential trend that they called it The American Diet Revolution. All the authors claimed authority and their celebrity endorsements guaranteed bestsellers. Cashing in on our insecurities, these books offered readers so much more than a few pages in a monthly magazine ever could. They created a following.

We tried everything from the Beverly Hills Diet to the Cabbage Soup Diet, utterly convinced one of them would work for us. But these diets were not sustainable for more than a few days at best, so we blamed ourselves, and our lack of 'willpower' when all our attempts failed. And in the midst of all this diet craziness, Jane Fonda stepped up with her fitness tapes, so we were now expected to do aerobics if we wanted to look like Ms Fonda.

We had been afraid of fat, but the Atkins Diet turned the world upside down! They said weight loss was all about achieving ketosis, so we peed on a stick every morning to check for ketones. They told us that high-fat, high-protein foods were good, and carbohydrates were bad. After all those years of deprivation, we happily indulged in the previously forbidden foods, gorging on butter, cream, bacon, eggs, salami, cheese and the skin of roast chicken. We may have lost a few pounds, but we looked and felt terrible – with bad breath, white-coated tongue, greasy breakout skin, and particularly unpleasant reactions in the toilet. Our bodies longed for all the vitamins and minerals we could only get from fruit, vegetables, and whole grains. Luckily, the next big thing was all about fruit and vegetables.

A book called Fit For Life encouraged eating lots of fresh fruit and vegetables, but only if we ate them in the morning. They said that we digested fruit and vegetables faster than other foods, so we should only eat them in the morning. The 'slower' foods had to wait until later in the day – like a highway, with the slower vehicles giving way to the faster ones. They made it sound feasible, and it was a simple enough rule to follow, but they had more rules about carbs and proteins. They called it 'food combining', which didn't allow carbs and proteins to be consumed in the same meal.

The Fit For Life philosophy seemed to make sense at the time, so the idea caught on, with lots of celebrity endorsements. The book was a bestseller. It hit American bookshelves in 1985, was published in Australia in 1986, and reprinted a staggering 24 times in the next 10 years!

We convinced ourselves that fresh fruit and vegetable juice every morning cleared out all the toxins and made us look and feel so much better. The electric juicer became the new must-have kitchen appliance, relegating the 4-slice toaster, egg poacher, yoghurt maker and waffle iron of the 70s to the back of the cupboard.

Thankfully, the notion of 'food combining' was soon forgotten. We weren't prepared to completely deny ourselves all those foods that broke the rules, such as eggs on toast, sandwiches, hamburgers, pasta with meat sauce, roast dinners, pizza, chicken schnitzels, or fish and chips.

In the 1980s, we were back to blaming the saturated fats in animal products for clogging arteries and causing heart attacks. This was a big opportunity for food manufacturers to ramp up production of vegetable oils and margarines to replace butter, and strip the cream out of milk. This phenomenon started in the USA, but soon spread to Australia.

It took years to gain traction across whole populations, but we were eventually convinced by our doctors, and incessant television advertising, to accept margarine in our shop-bought bakery goods and at our dinner tables. The USA had begun an 'industrial revolution' that created highly processed foods with artificial colours and flavours. Big corporations stripped the natural fat and flavour out of food, replacing it with substances far worse (sugar, glucose syrup, corn syrup, 'trans fats', and artificial sweeteners), and we were hooked. But it didn't stop there.

Under the guise of being 'healthy', we were being conditioned to accept vitamin supplements. Until now, pharmaceuticals were for sick people, but all these health messages had created a new market segment called the 'worried well' – people who were afraid of getting sick and were willing to try anything if it promised to make them healthy.

In much the same way as the diet industry was feeding our insecurities, the 'health food' industry did much the same. From a niche industry in pharmacies and dedicated small 'health food' shops, these corporate giants placed their products on supermarket shelves for people doing their weekly shop, who were invariably women.

In books, magazines and advertising, women were being told they could 'have it all' – a career, marriage, children, and leisure time too. But life became so hectic that we had little time for ourselves. If we were single women with an income, we were easy targets.

I can't name this weight loss company but they have been a household name since the 1980s, and have trialled many gimmicks along the way. They have improved over the years, but back then, their packaged foods were highly processed, freeze-dried concoctions and tiny frozen meals. If you wanted anything fresh, you had to buy it yourself, so it worked out very expensive.

In the late 90s I was at a low point in my life, and the weight was creeping on. I was desperate and easily coerced. I approached this company and was signed up for a Lifetime Membership which cost a packet of money back then. They worked on commission, and I was locked in. It was all a bit of a blur. It never occurred to me that a 'lifetime' membership suggested an ongoing need. Over the next 20 years, I kept going back to them again and again. I'd lose 10kgs and put it straight back.

I dabbled with Optifast diet shakes in the mid-1980s, when I was fit and healthy, but wanting to lose a couple of quick kilos for a special occasion. So, in 2003, having gained a stack of weight by then, I decided to try another diet shake. I signed up for the FatBlaster 3-month Challenge, hoping to win a cash prize for losing the most weight. I didn't win, but I did lose 20kgs, with a crazy combination of diet shakes, tablets and daily gym sessions. But once the deadline had passed and the cash incentive was gone, I lost motivation. I stopped using their products, and within a year, I had regained all of the 20kg and added another 5kgs for good measure! Are you getting the picture? Can you relate?

I forget how many attempts I made over the next 10 years, but my weight kept going up and down like a yoyo. I sought help from all sorts of professionals over the years – doctors, trainers, physiotherapists, psychologists, a dietician, and even a psychiatrist. I explained my situation but none of these experts had the right combination of skills to help me move forward. Each focussed on one small area of expertise rather than treating me as a whole person with complex needs. They all had different ideas and nothing worked.

Short-term diets create short-term results

I decided to find my own answers, so at the age of 50, I went off to university to learn about nutrition. I completed a biomedical science degree, an honours research year in health-related behaviour change, and a Masters degree majoring in health promotion and assessment.

Armed with all this new shiny knowledge and my own lived experiences, I was convinced that the key to healthy long term weight loss was **portion-controlled fresh food**.

So, in 2014 I tested this hypothesis. I signed up with a widely publicised home-delivery service for calorie-controlled meals with lots of fresh produce. They delivered to my door every week, so I never had to think about buying food or what to cook for dinner. I chose their lowest plan, at only 1200 calories a day, expecting to see the weight drop away. But after six long months, I had not lost any weight, not a kilo.

What's wrong with me, I thought. Why can't I lose weight? It didn't make sense. But then I reasoned that I only had part of the puzzle. There had to be more to this than the simple equation of 'calories in' versus 'calories out' that we were taught in physiology classes.

I suspected it had something to do with the power of the mind, as all my dieting efforts were so easily derailed when I felt tired, agitated, or depressed. Keen to investigate further, I went to another university and studied behavioural psychology, with a major in counselling and behaviour change.

In 2018, with five degrees under my belt, I pulled it all together, and just in time. By this stage, I was at my lowest emotional ebb and highest body weight. It was now or never.

Using all my research skills, and lots of intuition, I found the answers I needed to create a simple and nutritionally balanced diet plan that really worked. I became the guinea pig for my science experiments. I spent months testing every element of the plan, took photos of every meal, and recorded everything in a journal.

I lost 35kg in as many weeks, without exercise, and I kept it off. You can imagine how I felt. I was over the moon!

I'd been keeping track of my mood swings and depressive episodes too, but I hadn't been prepared for what I discovered next.

The initial test phase for the diet was over 8 months, because that's how long it took me to lose 35kgs. But when I looked at the data and started drawing conclusions, I detected a significant reduction in both the frequency and intensity of my depressive episodes. I felt like Louis Pasteur accidentally discovering penicillin!

Without those bouts of depression, I didn't struggle to stay focused on my weight loss goals, and I was much happier in myself as well. It was a WIN/WIN.

I am not suggesting I have all the answers, and it is misguided to assume a one-size-fits-all approach to nutrition will do any good, but I am keen to share what I have discovered. So, let's start by taking a look at some of the most popular diets over the years, and see if you can spot the dodgy ones.

Can you spot a dodgy diet?

No fat, low fat, high fat, low carb, high protein, don't mix protein with carbs, only eat fruit before lunch – so many crazy rules to follow, and so much conflicting information. With more than 1000 different diets bouncing around the internet, dodgy diets are a dime a dozen. No wonder we're so confused! Some are backed by real science and others have merit, but can you pick the dodgy ones?

Alkaline Diet (no animal products)

The Alkaline Diet is based on a myth that we can somehow alter the pH of our blood, and by doing so, we can prevent or cure cancer. Yes, cancer cells can proliferate in an acid environment, in a petri dish, in a laboratory, but that doesn't prove anything. Our bodies have built-in safeguards to buffer the pH to safe levels, so our internal environment cannot be altered, to become acidic or alkaline. Those who suggest otherwise fail to understand basic biochemistry. This is not a valid reason for removing meat, fish and dairy from your diet, and if you do so, you risk nutritional deficiencies such as osteoporosis, especially if middle-aged or elderly (Fenton and Huang, 2016).

Normal stomach juices are highly acidic at pH 1.3-3.5, the small bowel is acidic at pH 4.5-5.0, urine around pH 6, a healthy mouth has saliva at neutral pH 7.0, and arterial blood is maintained around pH 7.4 (Baliga, Muglikar and Kale, 2013; Fenton and Huang, 2016).

It is true that eating protein-rich foods will increase urine acidity, but acidic urine is a good sign that the kidneys are effectively ridding the body of any excess acid-forming waste. As urine is a waste product, it's pH can fluctuate, but is generally around pH of 6 which is slightly acidic.

Atkins Diet (high fat, low carb)

Based on a bestselling book of the same name, this American diet was hugely popular when it hit the bookshelves in the 1970s. It was the first to promote the notion of ketosis – a metabolic phase whereby, in the absence of dietary carbohydrate, the body's fat reserves may be broken down and used as a primary energy source, resulting in weight loss. What they're saying is that you should stop eating carbohydrates so your body will be forced to use its fat reserves as fuel. That sounds like a great idea, and so simple, but if forced to use an alternative fuel source, your body can attack the proteins in your muscles too, causing muscle wastage and organ damage.

Yes, clinical trials have shown how people can lose significant amounts of weight on these diets (Anton et al., 2017) but replacing carbohydrates with deli meats can increase the risk of cardiovascular diseases and internal cancers. Short-term success, long-term damage. Not worth the risk.

Calorie-controlled packaged meals / delivery

There are a couple of major players in this space, and they've been in business for decades. Some people do lose weight on these programs if they do enough exercise, but in my experience, the weight comes back very quickly when you stop exercising every day and return to normal food. I never lost more than 10kg in any one year on their plans, despite giving it a go at least once every decade!

I always chose the lowest plan, at 1200 calories a day, but I often gained weight instead of losing it! I should have been losing at least half a kilo a week, but it didn't happen. I thought it was my fault, that I was doing something wrong, so I kept going back and trying it again and again. But you know what they say: "Don't expect a different outcome if you keep doing the same things over and over." I blamed myself, but it wasn't my fault. It was simply the wrong diet for me.

Without a long-term strategy, lost weight will return

On these programs, I kept thinking about the next meal. Food was on my mind all the time. I had avoided biscuits and chocolates for years, but after eating all the snacks in these programs, I found myself prowling the shops for supermarket versions of their chocolate-coated peanut breakfast bars, pancake mix, ice cream and popcorn. And that can only end in tears. If you do lose weight, it can come straight back when you stop buying their products, and I'm sure they know that.

DASH Diet (low fat)

The DASH Diet is an acronym for Dietary Approaches to Stop Hypertension, and designed to combat high blood pressure.

DASH is a fairly conservative plan based on the official dietary guidelines, but with less total fat, saturated fat and cholesterol, and more protein, calcium, magnesium and potassium (Abete et al., 2010). The first clinical trials of DASH were conducted in America in 1992, and it has consistently been hailed as a heart-healthy way of eating. However, more recent scientific evidence suggests there is no valid reason to choose low-fat dairy over natural full-fat varieties (Chiu et al., 2016).

Studies have shown that those who follow a diet high in saturated fats and red meats, and low in fruits and vegetables were 11% more likely to develop depression, whereas older adults who followed the DASH diet had a reduced risk of depression and heart disease (American Academy of Neurology, 2018).

The DASH Diet might be well balanced, but it cannot be considered an effective weight-loss diet, with an average weight loss of less than one kilo after 4 months on the diet (Anton et al., 2017).

Detox diets

Detox is an abbreviation for detoxification, commonly used to describe a process of clearing the body of toxic addictive substances such as drugs and alcohol, because their liver is damaged and needs some extra help. These medically supervised detox programs are usually managed in a hospital setting or other residential facility.

But in recent times, the word 'detox' has been hijacked by legions of unqualified people promoting very suspect concoctions. They try to convince us that their programs, products, pills or potions will perform a magical detox that our bodies supposedly need, ridding us of toxins and cleaning us out from head to toe.

As silly as this sounds, even the most improbable claims begin to sound genuine if you hear them repeated often enough, and if you feel desperate. Even a person educated in the sciences could become convinced by some of their more elaborate stories, and there is big money to be had in this growing market.

Despite the plethora of commercial detox diets claiming to be 'weight loss' programs, I failed to find any evidence of even one clinical study saying they were effective. No surprise really, as so many users have reported nasty side effects such as fatigue, headaches, insomnia, anxiety, nausea, and shakiness after following these low-energy, nutrient-poor programs. You should not attempt these without medical supervision.

A critical review of the evidence surrounding popular detox diets found no compelling evidence to support the use of detox diets for weight management or toxin elimination (Klein and Kiat, 2015). The following paragraphs discuss their findings.

- Many detox diets involve excessive use of laxatives and diuretics, while other promote potentially dangerous quantities of certain vitamins, minerals and/or specific 'cleansing foods'.

- Extreme fasting can lead to protein and vitamin deficiencies, electrolyte imbalance, lactic acidosis and even death. And the unhealthy mind-set of 'detoxing' equates food with sin, guilt and contamination, which promotes an unhealthy relationship with food. If we already have issues with food, why make it worse for ourselves?
- Studies in mice suggest that such severe calorie restriction may be causing unnecessary stress on the body's regulatory systems, triggering binge eating and rebound weight gain once normal eating is resumed. Sound familiar?

The Martha's Vineyard Detox is a 3-week program where you are supposed to live on nothing but vegetable juice, vegetable soup, herbal tea, and specially formulated powders, tablets, and digestive enzymes. This American pseudo-celebrity diet should only be attempted under medical supervision.

The Liver Cleansing Diet has you drinking a 'liver tonic' of Epsom salts over 8 weeks, which will send you running to the toilet and risking severe dehydration. The food component is vegetarian, high-fibre, low-fat, dairy-free, and if you weren't sick before, you will be after this.

The Lemon Detox Diet, also called the Lemonade Diet or Master Cleanse, is a nasty 10-day program of salty water, mild laxative, and a concoction of purified water with lemon juice, cayenne pepper and tree syrup. And you pay good money for this? You cannot be serious!

Back in 1985, I checked in to an exclusive health retreat just outside Sydney, at Wallacia. Rubbing shoulders with the rich and famous, I endured a 3-day juice fast under full supervision, followed by a week of vegan salads. No alcohol. No coffee. No cigarettes. No phones. No television. It was a detox from the outside world. We suffered withdrawal symptoms but managed to get through it as a group. We relaxed our bodies and minds with daily aromatherapy massages, yoga and meditation, and I slept like a baby to recorded sounds of rainforests and whales. I was not fat back then, but I was stressed. I lost 3kgs in 10 days, which is no surprise when you don't eat.

In summary, if you rely heavily on pharmaceuticals, alcohol, tobacco, or heavily processed foods, you will feel better if you REMOVE those substances from your diet. Similarly, if you eat too much of something, such as bread or meat, you might feel better if you eat less of it or remove it altogether for a time. But when you REMOVE something, you need to REPLACE it with something better. Choose wisely. It has to be sustainable.

Select fresh foods that feed your body properly, not some crazy diet that fails to provide the necessary nutrition your body needs every day to keep your mind and body functioning properly.

Why waste your money on pills or potions that claim to 'remove toxins and cleanse the body' when your liver, kidneys and lungs have been designed to do just that, for free! But if you think your liver is not working properly, ask your doctor for a simple Liver Function Test (LFT) next time you have a full set of bloods taken. Better to be safe than sorry.

Diet shakes (VLCDs)

Exercise science tells us that for weight loss we must create a 'calorie deficit'. We can do this by consuming fewer calories, or by increasing the amount of energy we use, by exercising. But what if we can't exercise? What if a person is sick, injured or disabled?

Many doctors and dieticians prescribe nutritionally balanced protein-based liquids like Ensure to increase caloric intake for patients who need supplementation. In fact, Optifast, the original 'very low-calorie diet' (VLCD), was developed for use in hospitals under medical supervision for the morbidly obese. But things were about to change.

In 1988, Oprah's celebrity endorsement of Optifast and the Liquid Diet on her television show made 'diet shakes' an overnight success. However, Oprah it was later reported that after losing so much weight on the Liquid Diet her 'metabolism was shot', and after 2 weeks of eating real food she regained 10 pounds, because she wasn't exercising.

In 1980s Australia, Optifast was available from pharmacies with a doctor's prescription. Eventually, restrictions were lifted, and the subsequent ease of access and affordable price point proved to be a powerful driver in its ongoing success.

Long-term use can damage internal organs

Dozens of copycat brands have appeared on supermarket shelves since then, all containing whey protein, with added sugars, vitamins and minerals – promising to help you lose weight if you replace at least one meal a day with a shake. But only those labelled 'formulated meal replacement' adhere to quality controls set by Food Standards Australia and New Zealand (FSANZ).

Replacing one meal a day with a liquid supplement can be effective for some people, but if planning to use them as your major source of nourishment over a long period of time, seek medical advice. You risk damaging your skeletal muscle and internal organs if the powders are not medical grade. And like Oprah, once you start eating normal food again, the weight can come back.

FODMAPS Diet (low carbs)

This diet comes with strong academic credentials. The FODMAPS Diet developed by Monash University's researchers is a dietary protocol to treat Irritable Bowel Syndrome (IBS).

FODMAPs are particular types of natural sugars (Fermentable Oligosaccharides, Disaccharides, Monosaccharides and Polyols) that can produce gas and bloating in the large intestine as they ferment, triggering IBS symptoms in some people. The usual suspects include wheat, beans, dairy, garlic, onions, sausages, cashews, figs, mangoes, honey, agave, beer, and kombucha.

If you experience the symptoms of IBS, a dietitian might suggest a 'low FODMAPS' diet for a few weeks to see if this makes a difference. Then they will guide you through a slow reintroduction of these foods into your diet to determine which ones you can tolerate, and which ones are causing you grief. This is seen as a reliable dietary intervention, but following a strict low-FODMAPS diet over a long period excludes a wide range of nutrients that support healthy gut bacteria (Hill, Muir and Gibson, 2017), so be careful.

Gluten-free diets (low carbs)

Gluten-free diets are not weight-loss diets, but they can sometimes have that effect (Strawbridge, 2013) because people stop eating 'fattening foods' such as bread, cakes, pastries, pasta, pizza, and anything crumbed.

Gluten-free diets are intended for people with Celiac Disease – a medical condition caused by a debilitating sensitivity to the gluten found in wheat, rye, and barley. Symptoms can include severe abdominal pain and bloating, and cycling between painful constipation and uncontrollable diarrhoea. Many other people choose to go gluten-free because they feel they have a gluten sensitivity, without actually being a celiac.

Whatever your reason for going gluten-free, make sure you include other carbohydrates in your diet, such as vegetables and rice-based foods, as carbs will always be your body's favourite fuel. Did you know that your gut microbiota feeds on carbs containing 'resistant starches' and indigestible cellulose to stay healthy and function properly? We'll explain later, but just know that you do need some carbs in your diet. Choose rice-based products and coloured vegetables.

Intermittent fasting (time limited)

Fasting is not new. The practice is common in many religions, and all of us fast between 8 and 12 hours every night without even thinking about it. Intermittent fasting (IF) is a weight loss protocol that extends the overnight fast even further into the waking hours, forcing the body to use stored fat for fuel.

The health benefits of regular fasting are well documented. Numerous studies using IF have reported major improvements in metabolic health markers such as blood pressure, effectively reducing the risk of heart attack, stroke and T2D. And if you need further convincing, an IF diet that includes some form of caloric restriction can be very effective for weight loss, but can also reduce oxidative stress and promote healthy ageing (Gabel et al., 2018).

The **5:2 Diet** requires a drastic reduction in calories on 2 days of the week, but then you eat whatever you want every other day. Studies of the 5:2 diet have reported a loss of only 3-8% of starting body weight over a full year – which for somebody weighing 100kgs is only 3-8kgs (Gabel et al., 2018). Hardly worth the effort. Proponents say it feels good to eat less now and then, but most people tend to eat more over the 5 'free' days when told they can eat whatever they like. Yes, IF has many health benefits, but do not expect to lose weight if you eat whatever you want when you enter the feeding phase after fasting. To lose weight, you must consume fewer calories, and the type of calories are important too, but more about that later.

The **16:8 Diet** promotes fasting for 16 hours, but then you can eat whatever you want for the next 8 hours. It sounds like an easy diet, eating anything you want, but anyone battling obesity will never lose weight on a program that permits unrestricted eating. Even if you are fasting for 16 hours a day, you need to find a way to cut back on calories to make it worthwhile.

There are many other variations on this intermittent fasting theme such as reducing calories on 1-4 days a week or every other day, but again, the remaining days are free days of unlimited calories – which simply does not work if you're obese and struggle to control your eating.

Keto Diet (high fat, low carb)

Genuine ketogenic diets have been around for more than 100 years as a medically supervised dietary approach for treating epilepsy. In recent years, some small clinical trials have reported positive effects using ketogenic diets to treat other mental disorders such as anxiety, depression, bipolar disorder, schizophrenia, autism spectrum disorder (ASD), and attention deficit hyperactivity disorder (ADHD) – but the evidence is thin (Bostock, Kirkby and Taylor, 2017).

Modern 'keto diets' are not genuinely ketogenic, despite being low in carbs, high in fat, and moderate in protein. Ketosis is reached only when the body is deprived of nutrients for so long that the body starts to break down its own tissues for fuel.

Simply removing carbs from your diet will not put the body into a state of ketosis, because you are still consuming calories in the form of fat and protein. It is only after extended periods of fasting that the body might enter ketosis.

Trendy 'keto' diets are a re-hash of 1970s Atkins Diet

Lots of people are jumping on the bandwagon and making money selling 'keto' foods too, but there is no such thing. At best, what they really mean is that the food contains very little carbohydrate but lots of fat and protein. In fact, for a weight-stable person, the keto diet recommends a staggering 80% of all calories from fat and 20% from protein. These 'keto diets' should be called low-carbohydrate diets, but that doesn't sound trendy enough to catch the imagination of young people who are new to dieting.

While it looks like an extreme version of the 1970s Atkins Diet, the Keto Diet is not supporting the consumption of deli meats to get their extra fats; they encourage healthier options such as fatty fish, eggs, dairy, olive oil, avocado and nuts, but too much of a good thing is not necessarily healthy. If you consume too many calories, the excess will always be stored as body fat.

The Keto Diet was declared the worst weight loss diet of 2018 by the US News and World Report panel (a group of 25 experts in the health and wellbeing field) due to its ineffectiveness for long-term weight loss.

Lacto-ovo vegetarian (lots of carbs)

Lacto-ovo vegetarian diets (LOV) include foods such as dairy, eggs, vegetables, legumes, grains, and plant oils. They follow a no-kill philosophy, so they do not eat meat or seafood.

When comparing a low-calorie LOV diet to a low-calorie Mediterranean Diet (MD), an Italian study found that participants in both groups lost an average of only 2kg over the course of a 3-month crossover trial (Sofi et al., 2018).

Low GI Diets (low carbs)

The glycemic index (GI) is a database of carbohydrate foods ranked according to their effect on blood sugar levels, which is something all diabetics need to know. The lower the GI, the slower the rise in circulating blood glucose, which has seen a huge shift from white bread to whole-grain and multigrain which are low GI (Abete et al., 2010).

While low-GI diets can be a good idea for some people, having to constantly refer to the database is highly impractical.

Two studies of overweight and obese adults reported an average weight loss of only 4% after 3 and 6 months respectively (Anton et al., 2017). Not enough to make a difference.

Mediterranean-style Diets (unsaturated fats)

The so-called Mediterranean Diet is based on foods from European countries with coastlines into the Mediterranean Sea, especially Italy and Greece.

This is where people were found to have lower levels of cardiovascular disease, diabetes and cancer than other Western-style countries. Scientists focussed attention on many of the common foods, such as olive oil, tomatoes, seafood, red wine, vinegar, yoghurt and cheese, and they became known as the first 'superfoods'. This became known as the Mediterranean Diet, with manufacturing companies being quick to jump in.

The core elements are fresh vegetables, fruit, wholegrains, legumes, olive oil, avocado, nuts, fish, poultry and full-fat dairy products, plus moderate amounts of red wine.

> **Mediterranean-style diets are balanced, but do not help you lose weight**

While this sounds like heaven to the average Australian who grew up eating Spaghetti Bolognese with mountains of pasta, meat sauce and cheese, the true Mediterranean-style diet includes very little meat, much smaller portions of pasta, and lots of salad. It is a healthy way of eating, and with appropriate portion control, can result in enough weight loss to have a significant health effect.

A study of 89 overweight and obese diabetic adults reported an average weight loss of 9% (7kg) after 12 months, compared to 10% (9kg) on a low-carb version of the same diet. Another trial of 100 people reported an average loss of only 4% after 12 months (Anton et al., 2017).

Mediterranean-style diets are thought to be the best for staying healthy and strong into old age (Voelker, 2018). They may even help to improve mood and alleviate symptoms of severe depression in some people (Jacka et al., 2018). But these beneficial effects are not being seen in those who are already obese (Franquesa et al., 2019).

Paleo Diet (no grains, legumes or dairy)

This celebrity-driven and highly controversial diet is based on an unsupported hypothesis regarding human evolution and eating habits of the Stone Age. These so-called Paleolithic diets are based on an omnivorous feeding pattern (fruit, vegetables, nuts, seeds, grass-fed lean meat or game, deep sea fish, and olive oil), but without any sugar, salt, grains, legumes, dairy and potatoes.

A few small studies have reported improvements in blood pressure, glucose metabolism and weight loss, but calcium deficiency was an issue. Participants found it difficult to go without all dairy and grains, particularly when other diets produced similar health benefits without creating nutritional deficiencies (Pitt, 2016).

There are very few clinical trials of the Paleo Diet, but one very small trial of 27 overweight and obese postmenopausal women reported an average weight loss of only 10% (9kg) after

12 months (Anton et al., 2017), but those results are not supported elsewhere.

Protein pacing (high protein)

This is something often discussed in the gym, and misunderstood by most, so it is definitely worth a mention.

A protein-pacing diet includes multiple timed protein-rich supplements and/or whole foods. The calculations are key, and you need to understand how to measure protein, but you risk missing out on essential vitamins and minerals.

A small trial of 10 men and 14 women tested a calorie-controlled protein-pacing diet for 12 weeks. They consumed multiple protein shakes during the day and a protein-rich meal at night. The average weight loss was 10% (10kg) for women and 11% (13kg) for the men (Arciero et al., 2016). This is popular with body builders wanting to shred fat quickly while in training for an event, but beware, chugging too many protein shakes can make you fat very quickly too.

Protein does increase satiety (feeling of fulness) more readily than fats or carbohydrates, and may help retain muscle mass during periods of weight loss. It is also true that a balanced diet – with more protein than carbs – may improve body composition, facilitate fat loss, and improve body weight maintenance after weight loss, but only when you control your total calorie intake (Paddon-Jones et al., 2008) – and that is the tricky bit.

Chapter 2: Under the knife

This chapter offers a brief overview of weight loss surgery, but is only general information and not intended as advice. If you are interested in learning more about the surgical options, risks and benefits, please seek medical advice from your doctor.

Is surgery the answer?

Does bariatric surgery offer an effective long-term approach to increasing health and quality of life (QoL), or are desperate patients willing to try anything?

In 2013, Australia's National Health and Medical Research Council (NHMRC) released their Clinical Practice Guidelines for the management of overweight and obesity in adults, adolescents, and children, stating that **weight loss surgery** is 'currently the most effective intervention for severe obesity. For adults of BMI >40 kg/m2, or adults of BMI >35 kg/m2 with comorbidities that may improve with weight loss, **bariatric surgery** may be considered, taking into account the individual situation' (NHMRC 2013).

This remains their current recommendation to all medical and research institutions, and not surprisingly, many doctors are in favour of surgical intervention when their hospitals receive extra funding to perform these elective surgeries.

The number of 'primary' bariatric surgeries performed in Australian hospitals in 2005 was averaging 9 000 per year, and by 2014 this had more than doubled to 22 000 per year. In fact, the total number of weight-loss-related surgeries in 2014 was a staggering 124 600, if you include additional procedures for adjustments, revisions and reversals (AIHW, 2017). But is this the best use of those funds, totalling more than AUD $60 million a year?

We know that obesity-related health conditions can cause chronic pain, disability, and psychological distress. Self-confidence and self-esteem can be eroded, social interaction reduced, and a host of problems exist around employment. It is undeniable that **our physical and mental states are inextricably linked**; physical changes affect our mental health, and our thoughts can affect our physical health and wellbeing.

When caught in the cycle of pain and suffering, we look for a quick fix to make the pain go away. More people every year are desperately turning to weight loss surgery, and they are getting younger, but do the benefits outweigh the risks?

The average male patient is in the high-risk middle-aged category (45-54 years) but more than three-quarters of all bariatric surgeries are on **younger women (35-44 years)** who have not yet reached menopause (AIHW, 2017). As obesity-related cardiovascular disease only becomes a major concern for women after menopause, why are so many young women undergoing surgery? One medical reason could be a last-ditch attempt to improve fertility during their childbearing years, but to me, these statistics raise a red flag. Why are so many doing it?

Consider the long-term implications

The risk of surgical complication increases as we age, so I can see why surgeons would be happier operating on younger patients, but isn't 35 too young to undergo such drastic surgery? I suspect many of these young women feel pressured by those around them, desperate, and willing to try anything for the chance of a better life. But I seriously doubt that they truly appreciate the severe limitations this will put on their food choices, and the emotional cost of living the next 50 years with a surgically altered stomach and digestive system.

Those of us who have struggled to lose weight have been told over and over to increase physical activity and improve our eating habits. Sounds simple enough, but like all good advice, it is easier said than done. Perhaps we can no longer walk very far, let alone exercise. Or maybe it's the depression and anxiety that keeps us housebound and emotionally attached to food.

Our bodies gain weight so easily, but losing it can seem impossible. No wonder so many people embrace the dream that bariatric surgery offers; the promise of a quick fix that will solve all their problems; the magic wand that will change their lives. For tens of thousands of obese individuals, it might feel like their only choice, but is it the only way?

Very few obese people lose weight with the traditional approach of diet and exercise, so it comes as no surprise that doctors see surgery as a reasonable alternative. But how much do we really know about it? What are the risks? What will life be like after surgery? Can you cope with living like that for the rest of your life? Is it worth the risks? What do you need to know so you can make an 'informed decision' about what is best for you? Before making any decision, ask yourself these questions, and in this chapter we offer a little general information to start the conversation.

What is weight loss surgery?

Bariatric surgery is a highly invasive surgical procedure to mechanically restrict the volume of food a person can eat, and affects how that food is digested. Developed as a way for obese patients to lose weight without exercise, it is often called 'obesity surgery' or simply 'weight loss surgery'.

In theory, they should consume less food and absorb fewer calories, thereby reducing their risk of obesity-related diseases. But surgical complications are common, and nutritional deficiencies can have serious consequences. More than half of all patients must return for additional surgeries – for adjustments, revisions, removals or to fix other problems (AIHW, 2017).

Laparoscopic procedures account for two-thirds of all weight loss surgeries and half of all additional surgeries. These procedures are less invasive and quicker to heal than open surgeries, as only a few small keyhole incisions are made in the abdomen to allow insertion of the tiny camera (laparoscope) and surgical instruments.

Laparoscopic Gastric Banding ('lap band')

Lap band surgery has been around for many years and was popular because it offered an opportunity for a reversal if desired. However, lap bands had high rates of additional surgeries to rectify problems, so most surgeons no longer recommend it.

Common problems needing attention include band slippage, band adjustment, band erosion, blood clots in the leg or pelvic veins, long-term band failure, respiratory complications such as pneumonia, and damage to other organs. In 2014, more than 95% of additional procedures were recorded as 'adjustment of gastric band', and more than half were for lap band removal (AIHW, 2017).

Laparoscopic Sleeve Gastrectomy (LSG)

This procedure is permanent. It cannot be reversed. Most of the stomach is removed, with the natural bulge of the stomach replaced by a narrow gastric tube or 'sleeve' held together by a triple row of titanium staples. **This sleeve can only hold about 150 ml or half a cup of food (about 10% of a normal stomach volume).** These physical limitations can cause serious nutritional deficiencies and negatively affect a person's social life and emotional wellbeing. Gastric reflux (heartburn) will need to be controlled by acid-lowering medication.

For the first 10 days or so there is a risk of stomach contents leaking through the staples and into the abdominal cavity. This can cause **peritonitis**, a serious infection which could see you hospitalised for weeks instead of days. If the sleeve becomes too narrow for you to swallow properly, you may need gastroscopic day surgery to rectify. If the sleeve stretches (which is common in pre-menopausal women) you might need a **gastric bypass**.

Laparoscopic Gastric Bypass (ROUX-EN-Y)

The **gastric bypass** is considered the 'gold standard' in bariatric surgery (Salminen et al., 2018). In this procedure, most of the stomach is disconnected from the digestive system, leaving behind **a very small 'gastric pouch' with a capacity of only 30-40 ml.** The surgeon will then divide the small bowel, bringing one piece up to join with the pouch, and another piece to provide a channel for digestive enzymes – a bit like a plumber connecting hoses to a new dishwasher. But don't be fooled. This is major surgery, and any attempt at reversal is fraught with complications.

Food will bypass the area of gut where most nutrient absorption occurs, so daily supplements are crucial. In the first few months, you might feel unwell after eating – dizzy, flushed in the face, and wanting to lie down. It's called 'dumping' – where food intake causes a sudden imbalance in blood sugar levels (Weledji, 2016).

As with the sleeve gastrectomy, it is possible for the surgical joins of the gastric bypass to inadvertently leak gastric fluid into the abdominal cavity during the first couple of weeks after surgery – as the joins begin to heal. Peritonitis is a serious complication and may require 'open' surgery. If so, expect weeks in hospital and a stay in an intensive care unit (ICU). Again, in the first few weeks, swallowing might become difficult due to a narrowing of the surgical join between the small bowel and the new pouch, but this can be fixed with day surgery gastroscopy and dilatation.

There is a reported 9% risk of a hernia developing as a major complication, even years after the initial surgery. When the small bowel is resected and reconnected, there are two small holes that could cause part of the bowel to become stuck. Episodes of severe abdominal pain could indicate an internal hernia. If this happens, you may require 'open' surgery to rectify.

Surgical opinion is that any attempt to reverse a gastric bypass would be complex, technically challenging, and require major 'open' surgery (Chousleb et al., 2012) with functional success limited by how much **necrosis** (cell death) has occurred in the disconnected tissues since the blood supply was restricted.

One-Anastomosis Gastric Bypass (OAGB)

Known as the **mini-gastric bypass** or **omega-loop gastric bypass**, this less common procedure is gaining interest as an effective surgical approach for the severely obese – but surgical opinions remain divided.

The major functional difference with this type of gastric bypass procedure is the creation of a longer pouch than the other types, theoretically reducing acid reflux by keeping the bile stream away from the oesophagus. However, many research articles suggest that restrictive bariatric procedures (such as gastric banding, sleeve gastrectomy and OAGB) can <u>increase</u> acid reflux which can lead to cancerous cell changes in the oesophagus (Salminen et al., 2018; Solouki et al., 2018). Again, we have to ask ourselves, do the benefits outweigh all these risks?

All surgeries carry risk

All surgical procedures are risky, and that level of risk increases exponentially with how fat you are and the older you get. To consider those risks, we divide them into two categories: those specific to weight loss surgery, and those inherent to all types of major surgery. We have already discussed some of the specific risks associated with bariatric surgeries, so let's talk about some of the general surgical risks when we are overweight or obese.

Complications could include a bad reaction to the anaesthetic, infections in the wound or inside the abdominal cavity, breathing problems, blood clots in the leg or lungs, and even death. Excessive bleeding or the puncturing of internal organs such as the spleen and bowel can be life threatening, especially for those with pre-existing health issues.

While any anaesthetic carries a risk, the level of risk is substantially increased when the patient is overweight or obese. Some patients can have an adverse reaction to **general anaesthesia**, and obese patients are more likely to have trouble breathing while under sedation, so they might require **tracheal intubation** to maintain an open airway.

In 2014, adverse surgical events were reported for 7% of all bariatric surgeries performed in Australia, and the rate of 'accidental puncture or laceration' was one in every 100 weight loss surgeries (AIHW, 2017). These are just some of the risks, but you get the idea.

But even if you do decide to undergo elective surgery, you may be in for a long wait, depending on where you live.

You could wait up to a year in Victoria and 5 years in Tasmania (AIHW, 2017) or even longer.

Even if you decide to take the surgical route, why not try the HUNGER HERO DIET while you wait? By losing a few kilos you could reduce your surgical risk profile, and once you see the weight dropping away you might feel empowered to keep going and not give up. Surgery sounds like a quick fix, but can you limit yourself to only a cupful of food at every meal for the rest of your life? Are you willing to make these extreme lifestyle changes and face the prospect of serious medical complications? Do not take this decision lightly. You need to make a fully informed decision, eyes wide open.

Chapter 3: Reality check

Abdominal fat is a major risk factor for so many diseases, but we tend to ignore what we can't see, especially when we live in a modern world of comfortable clothes and stretchy pants. We stick our heads in the sand and say, "I'm ok. It won't happen to me". And when something does eventually go wrong, it is a complete shock.

As we age, our body composition changes, even if our weight stays the same. We slowly lose muscle mass and bone density, but we store more fat. Fat weighs less than muscle, so it can take time to register on the bathroom scales. Meanwhile, **visceral fat** is invading every nook and cranny of our insides, in and around our internal organs, out of sight and out of mind, until something bad happens.

Killing me softly

The percentage of obese adults in the population has doubled over the last 30 years. The average male is 7kg heavier and his waist has expanded by more than 7cm. The average woman is now 5kg heavier and her waist has expanded by 11cm.

But the most troubling statistic is that 63% of women and 38% of men had a **significant increase in their waist measurement without any noticeable change in their weight** (Gearon et al., 2018). What that means is that our bathroom scales don't always tell the whole truth, and our love of stretchy comfortable clothes is aiding in this deception. Before we realise it, we've gone up two complete dress sizes!

More than 5 million Australian adults are clinically obese, and 74% of these are aged 65 to 74. Disturbingly, it is rare for an obese person to live into their 80s or 90s; their internal organs are damaged, surgeries carry higher risks, and they have less chance of recovering after a heart attack or stroke. However, because the inner workings of the human body are so complex, **causation is difficult to prove** (AIHW, 2016).

An extensive review of published scientific data found an alarming amount of evidence for probable and possible causal relationships between obesity and some increasingly common health conditions (Franks and Atabaki-Pasdar, 2017). Below is a sample of their findings.

Probable causal relationship	*Possible* causal relationship
Cancer (colon, lung, kidney);	Oesophageal cancer;
Cardio-metabolic factors (blood pressure, fasting insulin, inflammatory markers, lipids);	Reduced grey matter volume in brain;
	Gall stones;
Coronary heart disease;	Cataracts;
Uric acid concentrations.	Kidney disease;
	Depression and other neurological disorders.

- We know that large deposits of fat can make breathing difficult at night, increasing the risk of sleep apnea.

- We know that every extra kilogram of excess body weight exerts an 8-fold burden on the knees with every step we take, damaging our weight-bearing joints, increasing the pain of arthritis, and restricting how far we can walk.
- We know that people with Metabolic Syndrome (abdominal obesity, insulin resistance, elevated blood pressure and high cholesterol) are at greater risk of heart disease, stroke and T2D (Abete et al., 2010; Ryan and Yockey, 2017).
- And we now know that obesity is associated with a range of mental disorders (depression, bipolar disorder, panic disorder and anxiety), and abdominal obesity is strongly associated with an increased risk of major or moderate-to-severe depressive symptoms (Zhao et al., 2011).

It is rare for an obese person to survive into their 80s or 90s

We can only speculate why some overweight people are healthier than others, or why people of normal weight get sick too. But did you know that obesity increases your risk of dying sooner than everyone else? Not only is your mortality risk higher than other people your own age, but your mobility becomes compromised too.

Simple everyday tasks like bending, kneeling or stretching become impossible, and you struggle to breathe when you sleep. These functional limitations can be uncomfortable, painful, embarrassing, inconvenient, and often quite distressing because your independence is threatened. These feelings can trigger anxiety and depression.

Just be honest with yourself. Get on the scales and calculate your BMI. Get a tape and measure your waist. Try on clothes that don't have any stretch in them and discover your TRUE body size. Accept that you need to make changes, and use these measurements as a starting point. If you can, try to keep emotions out of it. You can do this!

All fats are not created equal

Most of us are culturally conditioned to think of body fat as something unattractive and undesirable, but we all need a little body fat to survive. We need it to cushion our bones, to protect our abdomen from injury, to keep us warm when it's cold outside. Fat is good, but only in the right amounts and in the right places.

Our adipose tissue (body fat) consists of adipocytes (fat cells) which store excess energy in the form of lipids (insoluble fat molecules), and we have two types of fat cells: brown and white.

Brown fat cells look dark under a microscope because they contain lots of dark-coloured mitochondria (the power generators inside all living cells). These brown fat cells store lipids in tiny fat droplets and provide the energy for thermogenesis (to generate body heat) in cold climates (Duteil et al., 2017).

White fat cells are large single lipid molecules clustered together with other related cell types (stem cells, adipocyte precursors, fibroblasts, vascular endothelial cells, macrophages, and immune cells). Most of our fat cells are the white variety, and too many of these guys can cause problems. When we talk about losing weight, we are wanting to lose some of these big white fat cells.

Location, location, location

Our bodies prefer to store fat in a subcutaneous layer (just beneath the skin), where it functions as a connective tissue between the skin (epidermis), muscles and skeleton.

Due to its surface location, any increase in this subcutaneous fat layer is highly visible, and can make us look 'fat'. But we should be more concerned about the fat we cannot see, the visceral fat hidden deep within the abdominal cavity, in and around our internal organs (viscera). This invasive form of fat can interfere with the normal functioning of the liver, pancreas, intestines, stomach, heart, and other organs.

- Issues with the pancreas can develop into T2D or cancer .
- Non-alcoholic fatty liver disease (NAFLD) is a common liver problem, even if you're not obese.

The omentum is a large flap of specialised adipose tissue that looks and acts like an apron, covering the abdomen and protecting the internal organs from external injury.

All fat cells play a role in hormone production and regulation, and the activation of immune cells, but we now know that the fat cells of the omentum play a much bigger role. Due to their location, these fat cells provide a communications pathway for 'chemical messengers' between the organs (Platell et al., 2000). How amazing is that! But of course, if you have too much 'belly fat' these cells can begin to malfunction, sending mixed messages, which can result in those organs malfunctioning.

Yes, it is a tricky balance. The right amount of abdominal fat promotes insulin sensitivity, effective glucose uptake into the cells, and a healthy metabolism, whereas an excess of abdominal fat has the opposite effect.

Overwhelmed fat cells trigger systemic inflammation – implicated in CVD, T2D, autoimmune diseases, and many cancers

If we gain too much weight, the fat tissues suffer structural damage and destabilise. Pro-inflammatory cytokines are excreted and the immune system is triggered to initiate low-grade systemic inflammation (Scheja and Heeren, 2019) often accompanied by a fever. This inflammatory state spreads throughout the body and is the cause of so many of our aches and pains. Indeed, if we keep eating too much, the fat cells can become overwhelmed and cause the immune system to stay locked in overdrive (Lancaster et al., 2018). This leads to other cellular anomalies and serious diseases can develop (Lettieri-Barbato et al., 2018).

Abdominal obesity, insulin resistance, high blood pressure and high cholesterol – known collectively as Metabolic Syndrome – are the main risk factors for CVD, T2D, and many cancers (Masternak et al., 2018). Females are further disadvantaged by hormonal imbalances before, during, and after the menopause.

And you can forget about liposuction; it only targets subcutaneous fat, not visceral fat. Research studies have confirmed that liposuction has no effect on fat-related disease risk (Masternak et al., 2018). Dieting is the only solution.

Know your numbers

Obesity does not happen overnight; it takes a concerted effort on our part to consistently eat more than we need – day in, day out – for weeks, months, and even years! It can take years, if not decades, for all that visceral fat to accumulate in every nook and cranny of our insides, doing harm without us even knowing about it. When it hits, that middle-age spread has been decades in the making, and it's a dire warning of things to come. But if you're having a little giggle to yourself right now, maybe it's time for a serious reality check.

We use bathroom scales to measure our body weight, but as discussed earlier, we need to know more than just our weight. We need to know how tall we are, and the measurements around our waist and hips. But to do this, we need a few bits and pieces to enable the measuring and recording of our numbers:

- **DIET DIARY:** Go out and buy a foolscap-sized lined exercise book. This will become the record of your success, and challenges. Foolscap-size is best because you will need enough space on every page to keep track of all the food you eat every day, and any challenges you face, at least for the first few weeks. This is crucial to your success.
- **Bathroom scales**: Set up your bathroom scales somewhere handy so you remember to use them every morning, and make sure they're on a hard, flat surface so you get accurate readings. Make sure they have a

DIGITAL readout, but if not, go buy new scales. Get a reliable set, but don't waste money on fancy scales to measure how much fat and muscle you have, because they can't make those calculations if you're obese. Yes, that is frustrating, but it's true. Weigh yourself first thing every morning, without clothes, and record your weight in your DIET DIARY.

- **Tape measure**: If you want to, you can measure your waist and hips, then calculate your waist-to-hip ratio. You will need a flexible tape measure, available in the sewing section of most supermarkets. Another option is to take a long piece of cord, take the measurement, then lay the cord along a metal extension tape to get the reading. Your choice.

Record all your measurements in your **DIET DIARY**:
- Weight (in kilograms),
- Height (in metres),
- Waist circumference (in cms) (optional)
- Hip circumference (in cms) (optional).

Physical measurements	Baseline (example)
Height (m)	1.7m (170cm)
Weight (kg)	120 kg
BMI calculation (kg/m²)	120/(1.7*1.7) = 42

HINT: To visualise your weight loss, plot your daily weight on a graph. I used an Excel spreadsheet for this, but I've since found a few phone apps that are much simpler to use. A good example is an app called **WeightFit®**. Download it onto your phone and give it a go. By the time we go to print, there may be others, but this is a good place to start. We'll discuss this further under 'goal setting'.

Body mass index (BMI)

BMI is the most recognised reference for obesity, and it is something we can all do for ourselves. To calculate your BMI, you need to know your **current height and weight**. The BMI formula is your **weight in kilograms** divided by **height in metres, squared** (BMI = kg/m^2), but it is much easier to use one of the BMI calculators on the internet. Find one you like and keep using it.

Most adults are considered obese if they have a body fat percentage of more than 30%, represented by any BMI over 30. But if that's not confronting enough, authorities have now created additional classes for obesity, because more and more people are falling into this category. And the terrible truth is that most of us who are desperate to lose weight are in the morbidly obese category (BMI over 40), putting us at extreme risk of T2D, heart disease, stroke, mental illness, and cancer.

BMI	Category
Less than 18.5	underweight
18.5 – 24.9	normal weight
25 – 29.9	overweight
30 and above	OBESE
30 – 34.9	obese class I - moderate
35 – 39.9	obese class II - severe
40 and above	obese class III – very severe/morbidly obese

Muscle weighs more than fat, which means that body builders and athletes can weigh in the obese range without being overweight for their body type. But don't use this as an excuse; most of us are simply too fat.

But there is a slight reprieve for those falling into the 'overweight' category. Danish researchers are saying that anyone with European DNA should aim for a BMI of 27 instead of 25, which will allow for just enough body fat to be healthy (Afzal et al., 2016). As for people from Asia, India and the Middle East, recent research data suggests that their BMI should be set even lower than 25 to be healthy.

Whoever you are, BMI categories should only be used as a guide. Do not take it to heart if your weight pushes you into a severely obese category. Do not label yourself. Simply use that number as your starting point, and celebrate your success every time you see that number getting lower. Most of us will never get down to what they call 'normal weight', but we can definitely improve on our current situation, feel better about ourselves, and reduce our health risks.

Waist circumference (WC)

Body shapes vary between men and women, and between ethnicities, which makes this measurement a bit complex. Use the following information as a guide:
- European/Caucasian women should aim for less than 80cm, with anything over 88cm considered high risk.
- European/Caucasian males should aim for less than 94cm, with anything over 102cm considered high risk.
- Asian/Indian women are at high risk if over 80cm.
- Asian/Indian males are high risk if over 90cm.
- No safe threshold has yet been determined for Pacific Islanders or African Americans (NHMRC, 2013b).

Waist-to-hip ratio (WHR)

To calculate your WHR, measure around your waist, then measure around your hips. Then, using a calculator, divide your waist measurement (cm) by your hip measurement (cm).
WHR formula = Waist circumference (cm) / hip circumference (cm)

The higher the ratio, the greater your health risk. If it's greater than 1, it means that your waist is bigger than your hips, and that's a clear indicator of major abdominal obesity.

For example, if your waist circumference is 100cm, and your hip circumference is 120cm, the calculation would be 100/120 = 0.83 (which is less than 1 and a much healthier ratio).

Chapter 4: Diet is not a dirty word

By definition, a diet is simply a way of eating. As creatures of habit, we create routines by repeating certain behaviours. The type of diet we choose to follow is a combination of food-related behaviours and routines we have developed over time.

Our tastes and behaviours do change as we age, and at times we might question our food choices. This can be for any number of reasons – when training for a sport, to lower blood pressure, to prepare for surgery, to lose weight, or to feel better. But with so much conflicting information at our fingertips these days, and so many people sprouting opinions, how do we choose the best diet to suit our needs?

Know your nutrients

We need to eat to replace the energy our bodies use, 24-hours a day, even when we're asleep, and we need to eat a variety of different foods to enable chemical processes and cellular repair.

- Carbohydrates are broken down into their component sugars, with glucose being the preferred energy source.
- Fats are used to build and maintain the structural integrity of our cells.
- Proteins are broken down into the essential amino acids needed to build and maintain muscle tissues (skeletal, cardiac, smooth) and to produce the hormones and enzymes that facilitate all the chemical reactions the body needs to keep working properly.
- Vitamins and minerals are the assistants, the enablers, the tiny helpers that facilitate all chemical reactions.
- Fibre (soluble and insoluble) aids digestion and helps to keep our gut healthy.

Macro-nutrients

The **macronutrients** are proteins, carbohydrates, and fats. Because they contain calories, each is a potential energy source. Alcohol contains calories too, but with little nutritional value.

As a young adult, I thought of food in simple terms. I thought of 'proteins' as animal products like meat, seafood, and eggs. I thought 'carbohydrates' were starchy foods like bread, pasta, corn, peas, and potatoes. And I thought 'fats' were fatty foods like butter, oil, cheese, bacon, fried eggs, and the skin on roast chicken.

I thought all salads were healthy and anything sweet would make me fat and rot my teeth. This is what I read in women's magazines when I was too young to know any better.

They offered a simplistic view of nutrition, with just enough truth to make it sound plausible, but with enough nonsense to create strange irrational beliefs and behaviours around food. Sound familiar?

Many natural foods contain combinations of proteins, carbs, and fats

While it is true that animal products contain protein, they also contain other elements such as saturated fat, carbohydrates and fat-soluble vitamins. Plant-based foods are mostly carbohydrate, fibre, and water-soluble vitamins, but some vegetables are high in protein too (such as lentils, mung beans, edamame, green peas, corn, potatoes), while others contain fat (such as nuts, seeds, avocado, olives).

It is much more complex than I ever imagined, but many self-professed experts continue to spread the simple version because it does make it simple. But if you want to make good food choices, try to get your head around some of the basics. It took me a while to replace all my old ideas with new ones, but it is worth the effort.

Proteins

Our bodies need a steady supply of amino acids for cellular repair and hormone production. Complete proteins (such as meat, eggs, dairy, and seafood) contain all the essential amino acids that the body cannot make for itself without breaking down our own muscle tissues.

Vegans and vegetarians, who do not eat these protein foods, must learn to combine complementary vegetables, legumes, and carbohydrates (such as rice and beans) to compensate for the lack of animal protein, or risk major nutritional deficiencies. Beans and soy products are common protein foods for vegetarians, but they do not contain all the essential amino acids, so must be properly combined with other foods to achieve complete proteins.

Carbohydrates

Our bodies need carbohydrates. They provide the most efficient source of fuel for our body and brain. If carbohydrates are unavailable, the body can process proteins and fats into a usable substrate, but this takes time and is much less efficient. Carbohydrates can be 'simple' or 'complex' sugars.

- Simple carbohydrates are monosaccharides (single sugar molecules) or disaccharides (double sugar molecules). Glucose, fructose, and galactose are single sugar molecules. The double sugar molecules are sucrose (glucose + fructose), lactose (glucose + galactose), and maltose (2 glucose molecules).
- Complex carbohydrates are chains of more than two sugar molecules. Oligosaccharides have short chains of 3 to 10 sugar molecules, whereas polysaccharides have much longer chains of hundreds or even thousands of monosaccharide units strung together.

The healthiest carbohydrates are vegetables, fruit, whole grains, and legumes. The ones we should avoid, or keep to a minimum, are processed foods like bread, biscuits, and pasta.

Processed foods can contain unnaturally large amounts of sugar, salt and fat, to add flavour and a longer shelf life. When a food label reads 'low fat', the food will often contain extra sugar to add flavour. Similarly, if it reads 'low sugar' or 'sugar-free', it often contains extra fat and artificial flavours.

Natural sweeteners such as cane sugar, honey, and molasses can have a place in a healthy diet but should be kept to a minimum. If you want something sweet, reach for a piece of fruit.

Fats

There are three main types of dietary fat: saturated, unsaturated, and trans fats.

Saturated fats solidify at room temperature. They are found in natural animal products such as meat, poultry, seafood, dairy, and eggs, and in coconut oil.

Some years ago, animal products were blamed for arterial blockages and increasing LDL cholesterol levels in the blood, but more recent studies have rebuffed many of those earlier beliefs. Hence, many animal products are off my naughty list and should be included in a balanced diet – in small portions, especially if trying to lose weight.

Coconut oil gained popularity recently, thanks to clever social media marketing and misinformation, but the health claims are unfounded. The cultures that use lots of coconut oil also have extreme rates of obesity and type 2 diabetes, which speaks for itself.

Unsaturated fats may be a healthier alternative to saturated fats, but too much of a good thing will make you fat. These fats are found in a few vegetables, fruit, legumes, and grains, but the most common and prolific sources are nuts, avocado, and the oils – olive, canola, corn, peanut, sunflower, and rice bran.

Trans fatty acids (TFAs) are the ones you need to avoid. Tiny amounts of natural TFAs are found in meat and dairy, but the problem lies with the artificial form manufacturers create from unsaturated fats. These manufactured TFAs are used in industrial food processing, to harden vegetable fats in margarine, and to increase the shelf life of baked goods such as pies, cakes, biscuits, crackers, and pizza dough. Due to consumer demands, many companies have removed trans fats from their products, but check your supermarket food labels. Avoid, avoid, avoid.

Micro-nutrients (vitamins, minerals)

Micronutrients are the vitamins and minerals. They do not contain any calories, but are essential for all the chemical reactions that keep us alive and help us thrive. Importantly, there are fat-soluble vitamins and water-soluble vitamins.
- fat-soluble vitamins (A, D, E, K),
- water-soluble vitamins (C, B-group),
- essential minerals (calcium, chloride, magnesium, phosphorus, potassium, sodium, sulphur) and
- trace elements (chromium, copper, fluoride, iodine, iron, manganese, molybdenum, selenium, zinc).

Many processed foods such as breakfast cereals and baking flours are enriched with vitamins and minerals, but these chemical additives are not always easily assimilated. Supplements can help fill in some nutritional gaps, when needed, but they can place an extra burden on our liver. Our bodies are better equipped to absorb nutrients from natural foods.

Follow the advice of experts and aim at 'eating the rainbow' – fruit and vegetables of many colours – to ensure a healthy mix of vitamins and minerals.

Foods containing **water-soluble vitamins** should be eaten every day, or as often as possible, as the body can only store very small amounts. Many of these foods are powerful antioxidants and the B vitamins are crucial for our neural networks.

Recommended sources of water-soluble vitamins include:
- B1 (thiamine): Yeast, pork, cereal grains, sunflower seeds, brown rice, whole-grain rye, asparagus, kale, cauliflower, potatoes, oranges, liver, and eggs.
- B2 (riboflavin): Asparagus, bananas, persimmons, okra, silverbeet, cottage cheese, ricotta cheese, milk, yoghurt, steak, eggs, fish, oysters, and green beans.
- B3 (niacin): Tuna, beef liver, heart, kidney, chicken, beef, milk, eggs, avocados, dates, tomatoes, leafy green vegetables, broccoli, carrots, sweet potatoes, asparagus, nuts, wholegrains, legumes, mushrooms, and brewer's yeast.
- B5 (pantothenic acid): Egg yolk, liver, kidney, yeast, meats, wholegrains, broccoli, avocados, royal jelly, and fish eggs.
- B6 (pyridoxine): Chickpeas, streak, navy beans, liver, tuna, salmon, chicken breast, bananas, cottage cheese.
- B7 (biotin): Egg yolk, liver, salmon, spinach, broccoli, yoghurt.
- B9 (folic acid): Leafy green vegetables, legumes (beans, lentils), asparagus, spinach, broccoli, avocado,

- mangoes, lettuce, sweet corn, liver, baker's yeast, sunflower seeds, citrus fruit.
- B12 (cyanocobalamin): Fish, shellfish, meat, poultry, eggs, dairy, and some fortified soy products.
- C (ascorbic acid): Guavas, capsicum, kiwifruit, strawberries, oranges, papayas, broccoli, tomatoes, kale, eggplant, snow peas.

Our bodies cleverly store supplies of **fat-soluble vitamins** in our liver and fat cells, so we don't need to replenish them every day. But they are fat-soluble, so we need a little oil in the meal to help their uptake – easily achieved when eating meat, seafood, or full-fat dairy.

The heat of cooking or processing does not normally affect the nutritional value of these vitamins, so you afford to be a little creative with your recipes. But there are notable exceptions. There are fruits in this list that contain BOTH fat-soluble and water-soluble vitamins, so you need to treat them gently.

Recommended sources of fat-soluble vitamins include:
- A (retinol, carotenoids): Liver, cod liver oil, carrots, broccoli, sweet potato, butter, kale, kiwi fruit, spinach, pumpkin, some cheeses, egg, apricot, cantaloupe melon, and milk. Our bodies convert the beta-carotene found in carrots and other orange-coloured vegetables into vitamin A.
- D (ergocalciferol): There are traces in foods such as salmon, tuna, sardines, oysters, prawns, egg yolks, and mushrooms. But 15 minutes of daily exposure to sunlight on the skin can produce enough vitamin D.

- E (tocopherols): Almonds, avocado, eggs, milk, nuts, leafy green vegetables, unheated vegetable oils, wheat germ, and wholegrains.
- K (phylloquinone): Green leafy vegetables such as kale, silverbeet, Asian greens, and parsley are excellent sources of vitamin K, which helps vitamin E do its thing, especially with normal blood clotting and wound healing.

Major dietary patterns

There can be any number of reasons why people choose a particular dietary pattern. It could be cultural, religious, environmental, philosophical, geographical, or economic. It could be allergies or food sensitivities, or simply personal taste. As you will see, the major difference between them is their primary source of **protein**.

Omnivorous (all food groups)

Humans are naturally omnivorous. Our digestive systems have adapted to a wide range of foods – of plant and animal origin – so our bodies can thrive with any number of combinations. Meat-eaters do tend to weigh more than vegans or vegetarians (Clarys et al., 2014), but in many cultures that is seen as a good thing.

Vegetarian (no meat or poultry)

- **Lacto-vegetarians** eat dairy products (milk, butter, cream, cheese, yoghurt), vegetables, and grains, but avoid eggs, meat, poultry, and seafood.

- **Ovo-vegetarians** eat eggs, vegetables, and grains, but avoid dairy products, meat, poultry, and seafood.
- **Lacto-ovo vegetarians** enjoy dairy, eggs, and vegetables, but avoid meat, poultry, and seafood.
- **Pesco-vegetarians / pescatarians** eat seafood, vegetables, grains, and often include dairy and eggs. They avoid eating land-based animals (meat and poultry).

Vegan (no animal products)

Vegans are obsessive vegetarians. They follow a strict plant-based diet which is high in fruit, grains, and other complex carbohydrates. They avoid anything that comes from an animal, so to compensate for the protein deficiencies, they must combine the right foods to achieve complementary amino acids.

Vegans can easily become deficient in essential nutrients, especially B12 (Clarys et al., 2014) – which is crucial for proper functioning of blood, brain and nerve cells. If you don't eat animal products on a regular basis, consider a daily B-complex vitamin supplement.

Flexitarian (occasional meat)

This is my personal preference; a fresh plant-based diet with vegetables, fruit, dairy, seafood, eggs, and grains, with the occasional inclusion of meat. Also called flexible vegetarians, casual vegetarians, or vegivores. Might sound a bit too urban trendy, but this style of eating combines key elements of many traditional cuisines, especially those of southern Europe and South-East Asia.

Australian Dietary Guidelines

The National Health and Medical Research Council (NHMRC) published a set of Dietary Guidelines in 2013, from research at least 10 years old; research that focused on what had been the major health risks affecting middle-aged men – namely, cardiovascular disease (CVD), Type 2 Diabetes (T2D), and a range of internal cancers. Realising that some countries in the Mediterranean regions had remarkably low case numbers, scientists looked for answers, focussing on dietary elements such as olive oil, tomatoes, red wine, and nuts (Franquesa et al., 2019).

> **Full-fat natural Greek-style yoghurt features strongly in modern diets, for heart health, gut health, and weight loss**

The NHMRC used the results from those early studies, telling us to limit our intake of saturated fat, sugar, salt, processed foods, and alcohol. They recommended 30 minutes of daily exercise, a diet including all major food groups, and lots of coloured vegetables for their vitamins and minerals. They said we should eat more beans, legumes, fruit, wholegrains, lean protein, low-fat dairy, nuts, seeds, and vegetable oils (NHMRC, 2013a). This became known as the Mediterranean Diet.

Interestingly, more recent studies into obesity have found that full-fat dairy, especially natural Greek-style yoghurt, is much better for weight loss than all the low-fat versions (Bell et al., 2018).

Eating for your age

Everything changes as we get older, and that is perhaps the toughest pill to swallow. We were once fit and healthy, able to eat and drink whatever we wanted. If we gained a few kilos, we quickly lost it too. But those days are long gone. If you don't believe me, look in the mirror. Better still, take a photo of yourself trying to squeeze into those jeans tucked away at the back of your closet. Yeah, reality sucks.

"And yet", I hear you say. "What about all those who live well past their 100th birthday and say they have chowed down on bacon, eggs, sausages, pies, cakes, cream, chocolate, wine, or slabs of creamy butter on their bread every day of their lives?"

Yes, those people do exist, but they were born 100 years ago when life was physically demanding. Not us. We have electric dishwashers, washing machines, vacuum cleaners, heaters and air-conditioners. We can order everything over the phone or on the internet, without ever leaving the house. We drive to school, to work, and to the shops. No wonder we are so fat. But you won't see any really old people who are obese. Why? Because obese people tend to die before everyone else.

Our metabolism has slowed, and beneath our expanding waistline, large fat deposits have infiltrated our abdominal cavity, filling every available space. Simple tasks like bending, kneeling, or stretching become a chore, and our breathing becomes laboured. We start feeling old, and the thought of our own mortality fills us with… what? Fear, anger, disgust, dread... or resolve? Do we simply accept what is happening to us, or do we do something about it?

Calories and kilojoules

The energy potential of food is expressed scientifically as kilocalories (kcal), but most of us simply call them calories. Most countries started using kilojoules after switching to the metric system, but the USA bucked the trend and stuck with calories. Most nutritional databases originate in the USA, so many cookbooks and food labels display both units.

Australia's official unit of measure is the kilojoule (KJ), but I much prefer thinking and working in calories; the numbers are smaller, easier to work with, and easier to remember. I can keep a mental tally of my daily food intake if I only have to count 1200 calories a day, but I would need a notepad and calculator if I had to keep track of 5000 kilojoules!

Divide kilojoules by 4, to estimate calories

Keep it simple. **CONVERT EVERYTHING TO CALORIES.** But the exact calculation is messy – there are 100cals to every 418kj, or 4.18kj to every one calorie. However, you do not need an exact calculation. Nutrition panels only show an average estimate of the contents, so for our purposes, close enough is good enough. **Just divide the kilojoules by 4 to get an estimate of the calories.** It is that easy.

How many calories in a kilo of body fat?

Our weight fluctuates from day to day. A one kilogram drop on the bathroom scales can be due to an empty bowel and being a little dehydrated. Conversely, you might gain a kilo on the scales after a day of drinking lots of fluid, eating salty food, or eating meat that can take 24-48 hours to exit the bowel. None of those reasons have anything to do with losing fat. To lose a kilo of fat is much more difficult.

The energy stored in 1kg of fat is roughly 7700cals. Therefore, to lose that 1kg of fat you need to reduce your current food intake by at least 7700cals. If you want to lose 1kg in a week, then you need to reduce your DAILY food consumption by a whopping 1000cals.

How much is 1000cals? It's two frozen dinners, one hamburger, two pies, one and half bottles of wine, 4 beers, 500ml ice-cream, a small pizza, 3 pieces of southern fried chicken, 3 muffins, 5 roast chicken wings, or 200g bacon. Or it might be the calories in that overly generous bowl of fried rice or pasta, or the cheese and crackers and wine you enjoy every night. Even if you're eating a healthy diet, your portion sizes can be the problem. If you don't believe me, keep a record of what you're currently eating every day. It might surprise you.

To lose weight, overweight or obese adult females should aim to consume no more than 1200-1500cals a day, whereas males should aim for 1500-1800cals (Jensen et al., 2014).

Calculating your metabolic rate

Ok, here's something you don't really need to know, but it is worth mentioning just in case an overly eager personal trainer tries throwing these numbers at you one day. It is a theoretical algorithm used in academic research.

This algorithm calculates a person's **Basal Metabolic Rate (BMR)** – which is how much energy (calories) a body uses **at rest**, just to keep you alive and maintain basic bodily functions.

If you then add an estimate of how many calories you need every day to cover your physical activities, you know how many calories worth of food you need to consume.

There are online calculators that help estimate these things for you, but don't take them too seriously. They are interesting tools, but they can over-estimate how much food you need by more than 20%. The algorithm was developed using data from young male athletes, and it doesn't make any allowances for height, age, gender, or low levels of physical activity.

If you eat too much, you will gain weight. If you eat less, you will lose weight. Don't make it too complicated or you will give up before you even start.

Chapter 5: Superfoods – fact or fiction?

Everyone is talking about 'superfoods' these days, attributing some miraculous and often outlandish health benefit to the consumption of an otherwise very humble fruit, vegetable, herb, or spice. This chapter may not say what you were hoping to hear, but I ask you to keep an open mind. You might be surprised.

Marketing hype

Social media marketing campaigns continue to push the notion of 'Superfoods'. But should we believe all the hype? Is there some magical health benefit to drinking a turmeric latte, or tea with yak butter, by drenching everything in olive oil, or by swallowing coconut oil by the spoonful? The simple answer is NO. But if you believed all this hype, do not feel bad; you are not alone. These slick opportunists position their product in the marketplace by attaching a story to it that includes just a pinch of the truth, just enough to make their claims sound plausible.

Typically, these purveyors of misinformation quote animal studies to support their claims, implying that what happens to genetically altered mice in a laboratory experiment might also apply to humans, or they place a few human cells into a petri dish in a laboratory to trigger an effect. Nice try, but when it comes to nutrition, animal studies seldom have any relevance to humans, and those laboratory experiments fail to take into account the complexities of the human body (Crowe, 2018).

But we WANT to believe! We want a miracle, a quick fix, a pill or potion, not more smoke and mirrors.

Superfoods do NOT exist. There is NO reputable scientific evidence to support the notion that any single food can prevent heart disease, cure cancer, make us live longer, or help us lose weight! The 'superfood' hype is nothing more than a slick marketing myth, invented by people who either misunderstand the science or are pushing their own dodgy bandwagon for personal gain. So, what should we think about the latest trends?

- Freshly juiced fruit and vegetables have been popular for decades. They provide a quick and easy way to consume lots of plant nutrition, but beware of consuming way too many calories and missing out on all the probiotic goodness left behind in the pulp.
- The chlorophyll in your wheat grass shots might be okay for cows feeding in a pasture, but it doesn't do you any good just because it's green! There is no evidence to support the claims companies are making about wheatgrass, whether it's a juice, powder or tablet (Clemons, 2006). One ounce of spinach has the same amount of protein, but 20 times the vitamin A, eight times the vitamin C, and three times the magnesium,

calcium and potassium. So why would you swallow wheat grass?

- Coconut oil is used in cosmetics to soften skin and hair, and you can cook with it if you like the flavour, but there is no good reason to swallow it straight from the jar like a medicine! This saturated oil will quickly make you fat, and nothing more (Khaw et al., 2018). Cultures that cook with coconut oil have the highest rates of obesity and heart disease.

Most 'superfood' claims are wishful thinking

- And speaking of unnecessary oils, when did it become trendy to dip bread into olive oil at restaurants? It might have a place in rustic Mediterranean villages to fill up empty bellies, but do you really need the extra calories?
- And why would you want yak butter and salt in your tea? Remote tribes in Tibet might need to fortify their tea with yak butter to stay alive in their harsh climate, but we certainly don't need those extra calories, or an extra layer of fat to keep warm.
- And turmeric lattes? Don't get me started. Turmeric is the yellow colouring in curry powder, consumed every day across the Indian sub-continent, and yet those populations have some of the highest rates of type 2 diabetes. The active ingredient is curcumin, a polyphenol and antioxidant, but it is poorly absorbed, quickly metabolised, and rapidly eliminated. It has such poor bioavailability in humans that no health benefits apply. You would need to add it to other herbs and

spices containing the chemical element pinene (in black pepper, cloves, cinnamon, coriander, anise, marjoram, fennel, rosemary, sage, or myrtle) to increase bioavailability and enhance the release of any antioxidant properties (Hewlings and Kalman, 2017). So why bother, when so many other antioxidants do a better job?

Functional foods, not Superfoods

I'll say it again. Superfoods do not exist! They are a myth perpetrated by people who misrepresent the science. But there is a growing body of evidence supporting the notion that some foods do contain functional components – such as antioxidants or omega-3 fatty acids – which are known to provide some special health benefits. Others are thought to have a probiotic or prebiotic effect on gut bacteria. It is an expanding area of research.

The current recommendation is that most adults could benefit from including functional foods in a healthy balanced diet, and here are a few reasons why:

- Potassium-rich foods such as leafy greens, mushrooms, celery, yoghurt, potatoes, sweet potatoes, lentils and beans (lima, pinto, kidney) may help reduce the risk of high blood pressure and stroke by assisting kidney function.
- Polyphenols are found in many plant-derived foods, such as apples, berries, citrus fruit, plums, broccoli, cocoa, tea and coffee. There is substantial epidemiological evidence that a diet including these foods may help protect against developing cardiovascular disease and type 2 diabetes. Some of the active ingredients are

- flavanols (cocoa, tea, apples, broad beans), flavanones (hesperidin in citrus fruit), hydroxycinnamates (coffee and many fruits), flavanols (quercetin in onions, apples, tea) and anthocyanins (berries) (Williamson, 2017).
- Dietary inulin and fructo-oligosaccharides (FOS) from whole grains, beetroot, onions, garlic, honey, leeks, asparagus and chicory may help with magnesium and calcium absorption.
- Saponins may have a positive effect on longevity, and they are present in beans and other legumes.
- The pectin in apples might help reduce the LDL cholesterol produced by the liver.
- Rolled oats contain more than 20 unique avenanthramides (polyphenols) and beta-glucans (soluble fibre) that may help your body evacuate excess cholesterol that could otherwise contribute to blocked arteries.

Aim for a balanced diet... with seafood, greens, berries, and natural yoghurt

- The lycopene in tomatoes could play a part in reducing the risk of prostate cancer in some men.
- Isoflavones (a type of polyphenol) are found in legumes such as soybeans (tofu), chickpeas, fava beans, pistachios and peanuts, all common in Asian cultures which have lower rates of CVD and some types of cancer.
- Some foods exhibit natural chelating properties, so they may help to eliminate heavy metals – coriander, the

malic acid in grapes and wine, the citric acid in citrus fruit, succinic acid in apples and blueberries, the pectin in the peel and pulp of citrus fruit, and a type of green algae called chlorella (Klein & Kiat, 2015).

As an example, the following list is what a balanced diet could look like if you included lots of healthy and tasty functional foods:

- European and Asian cruciferous vegetables (broccolini, broccoli, silver beet, cauliflower, turnips, Brussels sprouts, kale, bok choy, cabbage, radishes),
- herbs and spices,
- rolled oats,
- unsalted nuts and seeds (walnuts, linseed),
- black or green tea,
- strawberries,
- oily fish and other seafood (tuna, salmon, sardines, mackerel, seaweed/nori),
- cocoa,
- soybean products (soy milk, tofu),
- tomatoes, and
- natural full-fat Greek-style yoghurt (Crowe, 2018).

Antioxidants

Our bodies produce just enough of its own antioxidants to counteract the normal production of 'free radicals', but lifestyle factors – stress, pollution, alcohol, smoking, or a poor diet – can increase demand (Adcock, 2018). When this happens, we need to help our bodies by eating foods with antioxidant capability.

The phytonutrients (natural vitamins, minerals, polyphenols, isothiocyanates, carotenoids) found in unprocessed plant-based foods contain the most powerful antioxidants.

- Vitamins A, C and E abound in many fruits and vegetables, such as carrots, citrus, berries, spinach, broccoli, and avocado.
- Foods such as shellfish, oysters, dark green leafy veg, black pepper, eggs, dairy, oats, and pineapple contain minerals such as zinc, copper, manganese, iron and selenium that help to create antioxidant enzymes in the body.
- Cruciferous vegetables such as broccoli, cabbage and kale are rich sources of sulphur-containing compounds that are broken down to form isothiocyanates.

Polyphenols are powerful antioxidants

- Polyphenols are a group of naturally occurring plant-based chemical elements (flavonoids, tannins, phenolic acids). Their antioxidant capabilities are linked to the catechins and tannins found in tea; hesperidin in citrus fruit; quercetin in tea, apples and onions; phenolic acids in coffee; and the red, blue and purple anthocyanins in berries, grapes, eggplant, and red cabbage. For lovers of dark chocolate, the bitterness of high-quality cocoa is due to catechins, flavanol glycosides, anthocyanins, and procyanidins. *Oleocanthal* is a polyphenol and potent antioxidant found in unripe green olives used to make cold-pressed extra virgin olive oil – but this compound is not found in black olives or any other types of olive

oil (Caballero, Finglas and Toldra, 2016). Polyphenols are thought to have a positive effect on gut microbiota (Jiang, 2019).
- Most herbs and spices contain bioactive antioxidant compounds (such as flavonoids, phenolic acids, lignans, essential oils, sulphur-containing compounds, tannins, alkaloids, and vitamins). They enhance the flavour, aroma, and colour of food and beverages, but they can also help protect us from acute and chronic diseases, due to their high antioxidant ability (Yashin et al., 2017).

Polyunsaturated fatty acids (PUFAs)

There are two major classes of polyunsaturated fatty acids (PUFAs):
- omega-3 fatty acids (EPA, DHA, ALA), and
- omega-6 fatty acids.

Omega-3 fatty acids

Seafood is the best natural source of Omega-3, and yet many people do not eat enough of it. There is another solution, but I need to get a little technical to explain. There are three types of omega-3 PUFAs: eicosapentaenoic acid (EPA), docosahexaenoic acid (DHA) and alpha-linolenic acid (ALA).
- The best source of omega-3 is EPA/DHA, from **oily fish** (salmon, mackerel, tuna, sardines, anchovies), some shellfish (prawns, oysters, mussels), and fish oil supplements. Unfortunately, unlike wild-caught seafood, farmed seafood are often lower in EPA/DHA but very high in ALA due to their feed pellets containing less fish and more grain, flaxseed oil, poultry and other

land-based ingredients (Caballero, Finglas and Toldra, 2016). That doesn't mean you have to ravage the oceans by only eating wild-caught seafood, but be aware that the nutrient content of farmed seafood will vary depending on farming practices in the country of origin (NIH, 2019). The cheapest option is not necessarily the best quality.

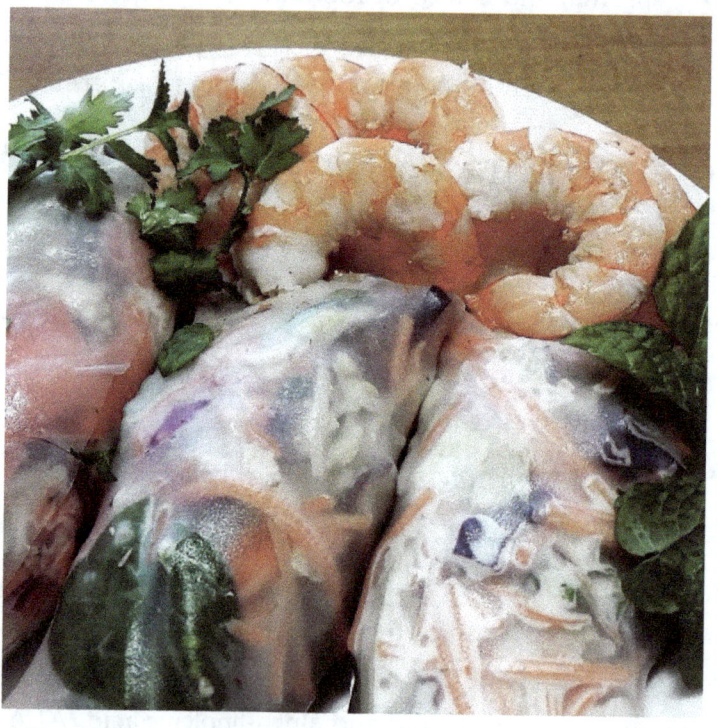

- If we don't eat enough good quality seafood containing EPA/DHA, our bodies can compensate by converting ALA into EPA, and then into DHA. But all this additional processing requires lots of extra vitamins and minerals to make it happen (B6, Vit C, niacin, zinc, magnesium).

- A few plant-based foods contain ALA, so if you're eating a lot of these vegetables, you might be getting enough nutrients to enable the conversion from ALA to EPA/DHA. ALA is found in flaxseeds, avocados, walnuts, some vegetable oils, cruciferous vegetables (such as broccolini, broccoli, silver beet, kale, Brussels sprouts, cauliflower), and some herbs and spices (such as basil, mint, oregano, cloves, marjoram). However, the older we get, the more difficult that extra processing becomes, which means that adults should be aiming to eat more seafood.

Why are Omega-3 PUFAs important?

Doctors have been prescribing omega-3 fish oil supplements to heart patients for decades, but that approach is changing. A Cochrane Review found they provided 'little or no effect' on CVD risk or associated mortality (Abdelhamid et al., 2018). However, the American Heart Foundation found substantial evidence to recommend fish oil supplementation for CVD patients AFTER they had a heart attack (Siscovick et al., 2017) because it seemed to reduce the risk of a subsequent cardiac event in those first few months.

Omega-3s have anti-inflammatory properties. They help to reduce the pain and disability associated with arthritis, type 2 diabetes, dementia, circulatory diseases, some forms of cancer, and the systemic inflammation associated with obesity. But more recent neurological studies suggest omega-3s might play a crucial role in nervous system activity, neuroplasticity of nerve membranes, memory-related cognition, and neurochemical synapses.

- Low levels of EPA were been found in psychiatric patients with major depressive disorder and DHA deficiencies were linked to depression, schizophrenia, memory loss and an increased risk of developing Alzheimer's (McNamara and Strawn, 2013).
- A subsequent pilot study treated deficient patients with a fish oil supplement and their results showed an impressive and sustained improvement in mood symptoms (McNamara, 2016).
- A large study of hundreds of patients in the Netherlands found those in the midst of a major depressive episode had much lower levels of omega-3s circulating in their blood (Thesing et al., 2018).

Low levels of omega-3s have been linked to major neurological disorders in humans

- Laboratory experiments with DHA-deficient mice suggest that omega-3 might be involved in maintaining the myelin sheath that provides electrical conduction for nerves of the central nervous system (CNS) – the brain and spinal cord – and provides protective insulation for those nerves. We know that any interruption or damage to myelin coverage can affect the transmission of nerve signals to and from the brain, but until now has only been evidenced in humans during autopsy of those who suffered psychiatric disorders (Le-Niculescu et al., 2011).
- In another intriguing experiment, with possible human adaptation, mice bred to seek out alcohol had their

alcohol-seeking behaviour curbed with DHA supplementation (Le-Niculescu et al., 2011).
- Omega-3 DHA modulates the same genes targeted by current psychotropic medications, and these findings suggest that omega-3 supplementation might prove to be both a preventative and treatment option for neurological disorders.

How to get Omega-3s into your diet?

It might look complicated, but there are lots of simple ways to get these beneficial omega-3 fatty acids into your diet, so mix it up and aim for variety. In addition to the fresh farmed salmon or prawns at your local supermarket deli counter, try adding 200g of wild-caught tinned salmon or tuna to your lunchtime salad, treat yourself to 100g of Danish smoked salmon and cottage cheese on crackers as an energy snack, or go retro with tinned sardines on toast.

Most major supermarkets sell packs of frozen wild-caught tuna steaks or salmon fillets individually wrapped in single portions. For a quick and healthy dinner, pan-fry or grill a tuna steak to medium-rare and serve with grilled broccolini or other greens. Or try sprinkling a few crushed walnuts across your morning oats or fruit desert, and top with a dollop of natural Greek yoghurt. Aim to include omega-3 foods every day, and you might be pleasantly surprised at how good you feel.

Omega-6 fatty acids

The most prolific form of omega-6 is linoleic acid, found in poultry, eggs, grain-fed meat, olive oil, canola oil, nuts and seeds. But there is a warning here. While omega-6 works well with omega-3, too much omega-6 can create an imbalance that limits the anti-inflammatory effects of omega-3s. Both the omega-3 and omega-6 must compete for the same vitamins and minerals – magnesium, zinc, and vitamins C, B3 and B6 – to become metabolically active.

> **Too much omega-6 can limit the effectiveness of omega-3**

- Seafood is best because it has more omega-3 than -6;
- Vegetables have omega-3 and -6 in equal amounts;
- But avoid meat from land animals, as it contains more omega-6 than -3, upsetting the balance and making omega-3 less effective (Caballero, Finglas and Toldra, 2016).

Prebiotics and probiotics

Over recent years, numerous studies have reported variations in the gut microbiota (bacteria living in the gut) in people with obesity, diabetes, liver diseases, neurodegenerative diseases, and some forms of cancer. We don't know why, but we have recognised possible environmental factors, such as dietary habits, drug treatments, intestinal mobility, and the nitty gritty details of how often we pass our stools and what they look like. Disease is often a complex group of factors, and we don't have all the answers. All we do know so far is that there are more than 1000 strains of beneficial gut bacteria, and people with certain diseases have more of some and less of others.

As the host, it is our responsibility to create the best possible living environment for our gut microbiota. To do that, we need to boost our dietary intake of prebiotics and probiotics. These foods are special because they can survive the journey through the digestive system to arrive at the large intestine where they are thought to be beneficial (Kovatcheva-Datchary and Arora, 2013). While our resident gut microbes happily feed on prebiotic foods, the live bacteria introduced to our intestines by probiotic foods may temporarily boost the numbers of resident gut microbes. In addition to the nutrient value of these foods, they work a second shift keeping our gut microbiota happy.

We have only begun discovering the role the gut microbiota play in our biological functions, but if we work towards keeping them healthy and happy, they might return the favour (Kovatcheva-Datchary and Arora, 2013).

If our diet is unsatisfactory, or after using antibiotics when we're sick, the quantity and variability of gut microbiota can be affected. Many microbial tasks will be compromised, such as the necessary breakdown of bile acids, the biosynthesis of B-group vitamins and vitamin K, and the metabolism of amino acids which are the building block of all proteins (Monash University, 2019). There are so many reasons to eat a balanced diet and keep our gut happy.

Prebiotics

Prebiotic foods feed and nourish the gut bacteria. These foods contain a special type of carbohydrate, a dietary fibre capable of travelling the length of the gastrointestinal tract (GIT) without being fully digested. These foods include a range of vegetables, fruit, and grains capable of double service, feeding both the host body and the gut bacteria.

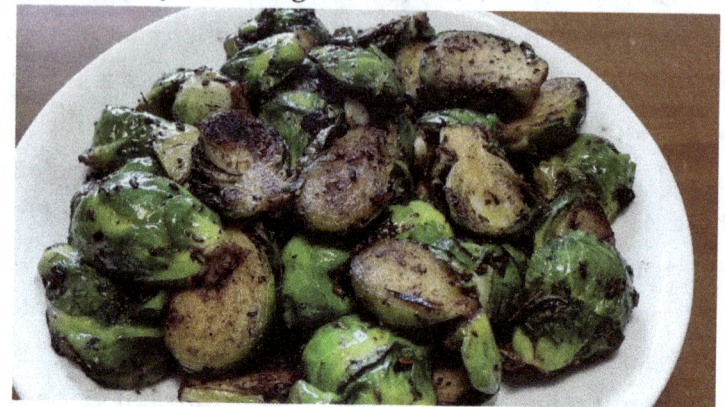

- Vegetables – asparagus, beetroot, savoy cabbage, onion, leek, shallots, spring onion, green peas, snow peas, chicory, garlic, fennel bulb, sweet corn, and the potato-like Jerusalem artichoke;
- Legumes – baked beans, chickpeas, lentils, soybeans, red kidney beans;
- Fresh fruit – watermelon, grapefruit, nectarines, white peaches, custard apples, persimmon, tamarillo, rambutan, pomegranate;
- Dried fruit – dates, figs;
- Breads and cereals – oats, barley, rye bread, rye crackers, pasta, gnocchi, couscous, wheat bran; and
- Nuts and seeds – cashews, pistachio nuts (Monash University, 2019).

Oats rate a special mention. They contain protein, fats, carbs, and are low in calories. Like other cereal grains, oats contain a polyphenol antioxidant called ferulic acid, but oats are the only grains containing avenanthramides – a powerful family of antioxidants. This traditional cereal crop is a highly underrated prebiotic functional food, helping to fight heart disease and colorectal cancers. Clinical trials have reported that as little as 100g can have significant short- and long-term health benefits – maintaining blood glucose balance, lowering LDL cholesterol and triglycerides, and assisting weight loss by making you feel fuller for longer (Li et al., 2016). Add a few oats to your diet whenever you can. Sprinkle a little over fruit and yoghurt as a dessert, or make a small bowl of warm porridge in winter.

> **Prebiotics feed and nourish our gut bacteria... helping to regulate appetite, sleep, memory, pain-sensation, and mood**

Probiotics

Probiotic foods contain specific types of live bacteria in sufficient quantities to provide a beneficial effect (Kristensen et al., 2016). But most products claiming to be probiotic are only fermented, and do not contain enough of the right bacterial species to provide any health benefit.

Even when a product starts off as probiotic, heat treatment during processing will kill all bacteria in fermented foods, the good and the bad. There is no evidence to suggest these products retain any probiotic capabilities.

- Naturally fermented cabbage sold as European sauerkraut can contain four separate species of lactic acid bacteria, but the heat applied during commercial processing can kill all the bacteria. It may not be probiotic, but sauerkraut does have other health benefits. Similarly, Korean kimchi contains lactic acid species but the commercial brands are unlikely to be probiotic.

Not all fermented foods are probiotic

- Kombucha is a fizzy drink made from a culture of yeast and acetobacter live bacteria, added to a base of green or black tea mixed with lots of white sugar (as the food source for the bacteria). There is NO EVIDENCE of any probiotic effect from drinking it, even if you make it yourself (Mantzioris and Deo, 2018). But tea is an excellent source of antioxidant polyphenols, without having to go through any fermentation.
- Apple cider vinegar (ACV) is an acidic condiment made by adding yeast to apple juice, with the resultant acetobacter bacteria triggering a second fermentation to create vinegar. As with kombucha, there is NO EVIDENCE to support the probiotic claims being made, even if it does contain remnants of live culture known as 'the Mother'. However, ACV does exhibit significant antioxidant capabilities.
- Many cheeses are produced through inoculation with bacteria and a fermentation. Cheeses that have been aged but not heated afterwards (Swiss, provolone, Gouda, cheddar, Edam, Gruyere, cottage cheese) retain their probiotic live bacteria.
- Natural full-fat Greek-style yoghurt contains live bacteria from the fermentation process, which may act as a probiotic.

Chapter 6: Who gets it right?

The Middle East and the islands of the Western Pacific report the HIGHEST RATES OF OBESITY, at more than 35% of their adult populations. They are followed closely by the USA, Canada, Australia, Great Britain, and a handful of South American countries (Chile, Uruguay, Venezuela, Argentina) (WHO, 2017).

The countries reporting the LOWEST RATES OF OBESITY are in SOUTHERN EUROPE (Greece, Italy, France, Spain), NORTHERN EUROPE (Denmark, Poland, Lithuania), and SOUTH-EAST ASIA (Vietnam, China, South Korea, Japan) (Science Daily, 2018). What are they doing right?

Southern Europe

The southern coastline of Europe, washed by the Mediterranean Sea, enjoys a unique climate with perfect growing conditions for a staggering array of fresh produce –

inspiring popular Mediterranean-style diets. From the sea to the mountains, each country has distinctly different regional cuisines based on their local produce.

Traditional foods include seafood (fresh fish, shellfish), full-fat dairy (milk, cheese, cream, butter, yoghurt), green leafy vegetables, tomatoes, cucumbers, herbs, citrus, olive oil, garlic, wholegrains, eggs, meat (mostly pork and lamb), walnuts, bread, honey, and red wine.

Fish stocks in the Mediterranean are depleting, but France and Spain, with northern coastlines fronting the Atlantic Ocean, continue to enjoy wild-caught seafood. Farmed seafood is becoming more common.

France

Classic French cuisine is famously indulgent, with rich cheeses, buttery sauces, wine, snails, lobster, and crisp baguettes. But the heart of many a regional cuisine is a hearty tomato-based bouillabaisse with local seafood – such as white fish fillets, clams, and mussels.

Greece

Greece is synonymous with barbecued octopus, souvlaki, salads, chunky bread, and spanakopita at street vendors. Lemons, yoghurt, olive oil, feta cheese, olives, cucumber, and tomatoes are everywhere.

Italy

Traditional Italian is so much more than pizza, pasta, and rice. At the very core are fragrant ripe red tomatoes, fresh basil, olive oil, and parmesan cheese. Italy has long coastlines into multiple seas, and seafood is characteristic of most regional cuisines – with squid, octopus, clams, prawns, lobster, mussels, scallops, and anchovies.

Spain

Traditional Spanish food reflects the Moorish influence, particularly the spices. Paella is slow cooked for hours over a fire, in a huge flat pan filled with rice, prawns, mussels, sausage, chicken, olive oil, spices, and chicken stock. Local specialties include Seville oranges, spicy red pimento, and fish (anchovies, tuna, cod, hake, herring, sardines).

Northern Europe

Europe's northern coastline is far removed from the mild Mediterranean. The chilly North Sea has a major influence on the western shores of Denmark, while its eastern shoreline shares the icy Baltic with Poland and Lithuania. Traditional foods are cured, fermented, pickled, or smoked, preserving them for long cold winters.

Denmark

Denmark produces some of the best smoked salmon you will find anywhere, but the traditional Danish staple is fermented rye bread topped with pickled herring, smoked fish or jellied meats, served with pickled vegetables, egg mayonnaise and a beer. White fish, lobster, prawns, and roast pork are also popular.

Lithuania

Lithuanians like herrings – marinated, baked, fried, or in aspic. Other popular staples include rye, potatoes, smoked pork meats, eggs, beetroot, turnips, mushrooms, horseradish, berries, and cold-water catches such as eel, pike, and cod.

Poland

Pork and cabbage feature across northern Europe, and Poland is no exception. They enjoy sauerkraut (fermented cabbage), pickled beetroot, dill pickles, sour cream, kohlrabi, mushrooms, smoked pork sausage, pickled herring, smoked trout, crayfish, and an array of freshwater fish.

Popular combinations include sauerkraut with pork sausage and bacon, roast pork with mustard, crumbed pork schnitzel with grated celeriac and apple, or stuffed cabbage rolls braised in a thick tomato sauce. The versatile pierogi dumplings can have a savoury filling (mashed potatoes, fried onions, white cheese, cabbage, sauerkraut, meat, mushrooms, spinach, cheese, duck, or lentils) or a sweet filling (cheese with cherry, strawberry, raspberry, blueberry, peach, plum, or apple).

Southeast Asia and China

Once referred to as the Far East, these countries enjoy warm Pacific Ocean currents. Extending southward for more than 14000km, the Chinese coastline juts out into the East China Sea like the full belly of a happy Buddha, continuing south past Hong Kong, to the thin coastal strip of Vietnam, in the South China Sea. The Sea of Japan separates the islands of Japan from the Korean peninsula.

China

The Chinese mainland is a massive area encompassing the full range of climate zones from the sub-Arctic to the warm tropical, with distinct regional cuisines. China is credited with inventing chopsticks and the wok, using salt to preserve and ferment food, and spreading the culture of drinking tea.

- A typical family meal would be a bowl of rice served with local vegetables tossed in a wok with a small amount of whatever protein is available, but other dishes could be braised, stewed, or even baked.
- The most common ingredients include rice, noodles, pork, tofu, seafood, duck, chicken, vegetables, seaweed, and soy sauce.
- Aromatic herbs and spices include ginger, garlic, star anise, cloves, chili, cinnamon, spring onions, black pepper, sesame oil, and fennel seeds.

Japan

Impressively, the islands of Japan have the lowest reported rates of obesity of any OECD country, and they have an enviable reputation for producing more centenarians too. In 2018, they had 70 000 people over the age of 100, with the oldest man and woman aged 113 and 115 respectively (Japan Times, 2018). Clearly, the Japanese have been doing something right for a very long time, but what is it? It could be a combination of many factors, but let's take a look at their diet.

Traditional Japanese food is light and full of delicate flavours – with lots of seafood, tofu, miso, rice, noodles, pickled vegetables, green tea, and nori sheets made from dried seaweed. Flavourings include soy sauce, dashi stock, vinegar, rice wine, sugar, and salt, while shichimi is a spice mix of chilli, lemon pepper, orange peel, black sesame, white sesame, hemp, ginger, and nori.

It is rare for a dish to contain meat or dairy, but fresh seasonal vegetables are found in most dishes. Processed soybeans are integral to the diet, by way of miso, tofu and soy sauce. Chilled rice-filled sushi rolls, wrapped in thin sheets of nori seaweed, will often contain thin strips of crisp vegetables with tuna, prawns, or chicken. Sashimi uses thin slices of raw tuna, whereas fish, prawns, scallops, and sliced vegetables are often coated in a light tempura batter prior to deep-frying.

Japanese Dietary Guidelines (FAO, 2019) recommend eating 30 different food components each day, with as much local produce as possible – including vegetables, fruits, milk products, beans, fish and rice – to drink tea, and to avoid adding extra salt and fat. A traditional meal consists of a soup with three small side dishes. The traditional way of cooking is with a light touch, by steaming, simmering, or grilling, to retain the nutrient value of fresh produce.

Unfortunately, the diet of younger Japanese is heavily influenced by Western countries – halving the consumption of rice and increasing the consumption of wheat, milk, sugar, salt, beef, chicken, and deep-fried food – all of which are known to trigger allergies and inflammation.

A recent 4-week clinical study compared a typical Japanese diet circa 1975 to a more modern version, and the 1975-style diet was a clear winner. The group on the more traditional 1975-style diet lost weight and improved their health. They experienced a significant <u>decrease</u> in BMI, fat mass, glycated haemoglobin (HbA1c, diabetes risk), C-reactive protein (CRP, an inflammatory marker), and LDL-C (the 'bad' cholesterol), with a significant <u>increase</u> in HDL-C (the 'good' cholesterol) (Asano et al., 2019). Compared to a typical modern Japanese diet, the healthier 1975-style diet had:

- more variety in fresh produce,
- more frequent use of simmering and steaming,
- more frequent use of soy products, fish, shellfish, vegetables, fruits, green tea, seaweed, mushrooms,
- more frequent use of soups and fermented seasonings (soy sauce, miso, vinegar, mirin, and sake), and
- more frequent use of rice and miso soup.
- moderate use of eggs, dairy and meat, with sugar and salt used sparingly (Asano et al., 2019).

Korea

Korean foods have stronger flavours than those of Japan, and their cooking styles differ too. Korean food is centred around grilled meat, seafood, and vegetables, with kimchi (a spicy mix of fermented cabbage and other vegetables, heavily spiced with red pepper, garlic, ginger, shrimp paste) a staple of every Korean's daily diet.

Every meal includes rice or noodles with lots of vegetables (such as eggplant or bean sprouts, heavily seasoned with garlic, red pepper and ginger). Octopus, eel, prawns, crab, squid, and fish are found on grill plates or in stews. Bulgogi is a dish of grilled beef strips marinated in soy sauce, sesame oil, wine, onions, ginger, garlic, sugar, and black pepper.

Korean cuisine is based on the five elements of earth, metal, fire, water, and wood – aiming for a balance between salty, bitter, hot, sweet, and sour. They enjoy fresh, pickled, and fermented foods, with popular sauces from fermented soybean or pepper paste. Ingredients in Korean cooking include:

- rice, noodles,
- sautéed or shredded vegetables, pickled cabbage, mushrooms, sweet potato, pumpkin, carrots,

- meat (pork, beef, chicken), tofu
- seafood (tuna, oysters, shrimp, squid, and clams),
- fried or boiled eggs,
- sesame oil, soy sauce, ground black pepper, cinnamon, honey, brown sugar, sweet-pickled radish, seaweed, soybeans, and lots of hot chili paste,
- fresh fruit provides sweet relief, with cherries, persimmons, figs, strawberries, melon, and apples.

Vietnam

Vietnam is a thin strip of land running north to south, with Laos and Cambodia to the west, and an eastern coastline dipping its toes into the South China Sea. Many rivers cross Vietnam on their way to the ocean, with the sprawling Mekong Delta to the south. Tea is an ideal crop for the highlands, while the sub-tropical lowlands provide abundant supplies of vegetables and seafood.

The cooking methods might look Chinese, but they use less oil, less meat, and rarely include a stir-fry sauce.

- A careful balance of sweet, sour, bitter, and salty is achieved with flavourings such as garlic, chili, cinnamon, ginger, shallot, lemon grass, fish sauce, soy sauce, lime juice, vinegar and sugar.
- Nuoc cham is a favourite table sauce – a combination of fish sauce, lime juice or vinegar, sugar, water, garlic, chili, plus shredded cabbage, carrots, or green papaya.
- Staples include fish, prawns, rice, green vegetables, fresh herbs, tea, and fruit.

Many dishes incorporate rice noodles. Some are served dry like a salad, while others are constructed using a master stock or broth to produce a soup bowl.

- Bun cha is grilled pork served in a bowl over thin rice noodles, sweet-sour sauce, fresh lettuce, vegetables, and herbs.
- Pho is the quintessential Vietnamese soup; made from an aromatic 'master stock' of beef and chicken bones simmered with onion, ginger, star anise and cinnamon; served in a bowl with rice noodles and a little protein (meat, seafood, or tofu). Usually accompanied by lemon wedges, bean sprouts, coriander, basil, mint, chili, and a bottle of fish sauce.
- Meat and poultry are used in stir-fries or marinated in lemon grass, garlic, and chili before being grilled.
- Leafy greens are often lightly cooked in a hot wok or added to soups at the last minute, whereas root vegetables like kohlrabi, sweet potato, ginger and bamboo shoots are often fermented or pickled.
- Seafood is plentiful. Fish can be braised or stewed. Fresh prawns are ideal for salads.
- Rice paper rolls are a popular street food of fresh prawns and shredded vegetables, wrapped in thin translucent rounds of rice paper.
- Sub-tropical fruits are abundant – longan, lychee, mango, citrus (mandarin, orange, pomelo, lime), rambutan, dragon fruit, durian, pineapple, papaya, watermelon, coconut, persimmon, strawberry, banana, passionfruit, avocado, plum, guava, pomegranate, apple, grape, and tamarind.

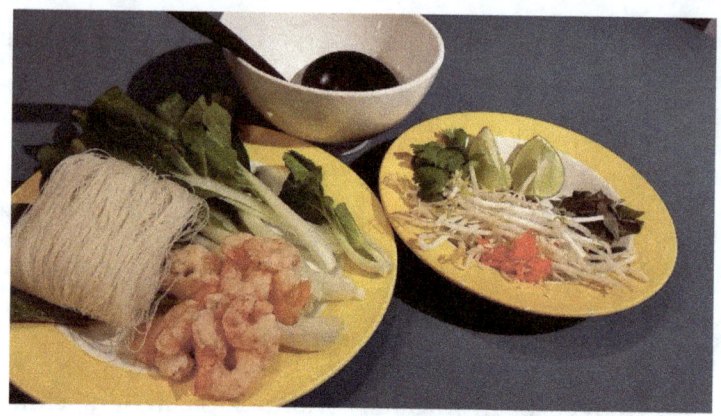

Traditional foods hold the key

Despite their diverse cultures, the countries with the lowest rates of obesity have much in common:
- Fermentation and pickling are traditional methods of preserving seasonal produce and retaining nutritional value.
- With coastlines dipping into multiple seas, they have some of the highest per capita consumption of seafood (Caballero, Finglas and Toldra, 2016).
- Pork is the primary meat source across Northern/Central Europe and in SE Asia. Other meats – lamb, goat, beef, chicken, duck – are common around the Mediterranean and in some parts of Asia.
- Eggs are a readily available protein source in most countries.
- Cruciferous vegetables are prolific and varied across Europe and Asia, and with more than 400 varieties sharing common ancestry.
- Popular fruits include apples, citrus, and berries, with tomatoes in Europe.

- Legumes such as beans, peas and lentils are popular across Europe, with soybean products in Asia.
- Some form of starch accompanies most dishes, usually potatoes or a grain (such as rice, pasta, noodles, semolina, or bread).
- Herbs and spices are added to European dishes as they cook, whereas in SE Asia they are often added to the finished dish.
- Tea drinking is an integral part of life across most of Asia, and more variety than in Europe. Herbal teas (tisanes) are popular in most countries as a caffeine-free alternative, but coffee is very popular in Europe.

Dairy

In Europe, milk from a variety of animals is fermented to create yoghurt, kefir, sour cream, and cheese, but this is quite rare in SE Asia.

Traditionally fermented milk products are probiotic, and an excellent source of animal protein, calcium, vitamins B2, B12, potassium, and magnesium.

- Yoghurt is by far the most reliable source of probiotic bacteria. It is readily accessible and inexpensive, often added to breakfast muesli or fruit desserts, but equally at home as a creamy salad dressing for savoury foods. Naturally fermented full-fat Greek-style yoghurt is made from whole milk that has undergone fermentation with a lactobacillus starter culture that feeds on the lactose sugars in the milk. Most adults are lactose-intolerant to some degree because we lack the enzymes needed to digest the lactose, but we can usually eat a small serve of yoghurt every day without feeling sick because most of the lactose is gone.

Countries with low obesity rates enjoy seafood, pork, vegetables, legumes, fruit, herbs, spices, tea, and fermented foods

- Kefir is a thick fizzy drink made traditionally in eastern Europe by fermenting milk (goat, cow, sheep or camel) with yeast, acetic acid and multiple strains of lactobacillus. As with natural yoghurt, the fermentation process reduces the amount of lactose in the final product, making it more digestible (Putta et al., 2018). Tibetan kefir has found its way to mainland China, but dairy products are a very new addition to Asian diets.
- Cheese is an excellent source of protein and calcium. Many European hard cheeses have probiotic potential (feta, parmesan, Swiss, Gruyere, Gouda, Edam, cheddar). SE Asia is not known for their cheese, but there are a few traditional ones (Chinese rushan, Philippine kesong puti, Tibetan chura kampo from yak's milk, Chinese nguri, Indonesian dangke from buffalo or cow milk, Japanese Sakura, Korean imsil).

Eggs

Eggs are an affordable and readily accessible foodstuff in most countries, especially SE Asia. Whole eggs are a complete protein, rich in B vitamins, choline, selenium, vitamin A, iron, and phosphorus, and they contain two potent antioxidants (zeaxanthin, lutein).

In northern Europe, egg mayonnaise is an accompaniment to plates of pickled vegetables with braised pork.

In Vietnamese street food, egg mayonnaise is a spread on banh mi, pork chops are often served with a fried egg on top, and there are large vegetable omelettes. Many Vietnamese foods show the French influence.

Fruit

Apples (Malus domestica) are rich in antioxidant polyphenols (Caballero, Finglas and Toldra, 2016), eaten fresh or processed into products like apple sauce or apple cider vinegar (ACV). China is the largest apple producer.

Berries contain vitamins, minerals, fibre, and a powerhouse of antioxidants (anthocyanins, phenolic acids, stilbenes, tannins, carotenoids). Most recognisable are the blackberry, blueberry, cranberry, raspberry, and strawberry, but Kiwi fruit is a berry too, originally from China.

Citrus fruit (lemons, limes, oranges, mandarins, etc) are popular across most regions and are prized for their vitamin C, folic acid, and other bioactive phytochemicals (limonoids, flavonoids).

Tomatoes are a fruit with vitamin C, and they feature in most Mediterranean salads and as a base for rustic sauces across Europe.

Herbs, spices, condiments

Herbs and spices are in abundant use across Europe and Asia. Oregano, marjoram, coriander, rosemary, thyme, sage, parsley, dill, mint, to name a few, and many varieties of basil.

Many popular herbs and spices – such as rosemary, sage, oregano, clove, and cinnamon – contain bioactive elements with antioxidant and anti-inflammatory properties that have a positive effect on gut microbiota, brain cells, cognition, and mood (Jiang, 2019). Salt, pepper, vinegar, mustard, and honey are popular across most regions, with soy and fish sauces in SE Asia.

Vinegars are made by subjecting fresh fruit to a double fermentation process – producing acetic acid, which is easily absorbed, readily transformed in the liver, and metabolized. They are used as condiments and to pickle seasonal vegetables.

- The French dress salad greens with vinaigrette – an emulsion of wine vinegar and olive oil.
- An Italian tomato salad is enhanced by a splash of Balsamic vinegar – made from the second fermentation of red wine.
- Apple cider vinegar (ACV) comes from apples treated to a double fermentation. In Japan, China and Korea, ACV is a popular folk remedy and taken daily as a tonic. Japanese studies suggest it may help with losing weight, maintaining healthy blood sugar levels, and lowering cholesterol (Kondo et al., 2009).

Legumes

Legumes are a class of plant foods made up of beans (including soy), lentils, peas, peanuts, and alfalfa. They are a rich source of B vitamins, minerals, protein, and fibre. Many types of beans are eaten across Europe, in salads and stews, while soybean products are synonymous with Asian food.

Fresh soybeans (edamame) are popular in Japan. Fermented soybeans are the basis for tempeh, soy sauce, Japanese miso and Korean soybean paste. Some brands of soy milk are derived from a ferment, but most soy milk and tofu are produced without fermentation.

Soy milk is a good source of protein, vitamin A, vitamin B-12, potassium, and isoflavones, with commercial brands often fortified with calcium and vitamin D. Tofu (bean curd) is a valuable protein source (with 9 essential amino acids), and important vitamins and minerals (iron, calcium, magnesium, copper, zinc, vitamin B1, manganese, selenium, phosphorous).

Meat

Pork is a quality protein, high in thiamine, iron and B12, and low in salt. Different cuts of meat and feeding practices can alter the composition of an animal product, but estimates suggest that minced pork or loin pork has fewer calories than beef steak.

Plant-derived oils

Nuts, seeds, and their oils are high in calories but nutrient dense. They contain vitamins and minerals (B-group, folate, vit E, calcium, iron, zinc, potassium, magnesium), trace elements (selenium, manganese, copper), plant sterols, and other phytochemicals (flavonoids, resveratrol).

- Southern Europe is synonymous with olive oil, walnuts, pistachios, and pine nuts. Olive oil, especially extra virgin olive oil (EVOO), is a source of monounsaturated fats, and polyphenols.

- Walnuts are rich in alpha linoleic acid, a natural plant-derived omega-3 fatty acid. Chestnuts and hazelnuts are across northern Europe and into China.
- Sesame seeds are hugely popular through Greece, Germany, Poland, France, and Italy, while the seeds and the oil are both used in Asian cooking.
- Peanuts are not true nuts, but most Asian cooking starts with a splash of poly-unsaturated peanut oil into a hot wok.
- French vinaigrette is oil and vinegar; mayonnaise is an emulsion of egg yolks, oil, vinegar, mustard powder, and salt.

Seafood

With access to so many rivers and oceans, SE Asia and the countries of northern and southern Europe use many different varieties of seafood in their diet. It is a high quality, low fat, low-calorie protein food, and a major source of iodine, selenium, vitamins B12 and D, and omega-3s.

Seafood includes all types of finned fish (such as cod, salmon, tuna) and shellfish (crustacea and molluscs) - eaten raw, soused in lemon juice, grilled, smoked, pickled, or immersed in a boiling liquid.

- Crustacea have jointed legs, a hard shell and no backbone (crabs, crayfish, lobsters, prawns, shrimp).
- Most molluscs have a hinged two-part shell (clams, mussels, oysters, scallops) but others do not (octopus, snails, squid).
- Salmon, tuna and mackerel all contain omega-3 PUFA and vitamin B12, and so do herrings, sardines and seaweed. Salmon and tuna both contain vitamins B3,

B12, D and phosphorus. Canned salmon provides calcium if you mash up the soft bones and eat them too.

- Sardines are rich in iron, selenium and calcium. Anchovies provide iron and zinc.
- White fish such as barramundi, hake, cod, snapper, whiting are an excellent source of B6, B12, magnesium and potassium, and lower in calories because they contain less omega-3 oils than fatty fish like salmon and tuna.
- Nori are crisp edible sheets of dried seaweed (red algae) used to wrap Japanese sushi rolls or add to miso soup. Seaweed is a good source of iodine, potassium, magnesium, calcium, iron, zinc, vitamins A, C, B12 and other trace elements.

Teas and tisanes

There are many types of tea – white, green, oolong, black – made from the leaves or buds of the tea plant (camellia sinensis). They all have some level of caffeine and are a rich source of antioxidant polyphenols.

Herbal teas are not real teas, but tisanes – hot water infusions of herbs or other organic matter (peppermint, camomile, licorice, rose hip, ginger, sage, etc). They do not contain any of the caffeine or antioxidant polyphenols present in tea leaves, but the herbs and spices being infused may have some recognised health benefits.

Many European and SE Asian countries add culinary herbs and spices to their teas and tisanes, as traditional folk remedies for digestive or breathing issues. Infusions may be individual herbs or a combination of spices – chili pepper, cinnamon, ginger, black pepper, turmeric, fenugreek, rosemary, garlic, cardamom, coriander, mint, parsley, turmeric, sage, rose hip, licorice, peppermint, camomile, fennel.

- Tea ceremonies across SE Asia (China, Japan, Korea) show the importance of tea in those traditional cultures.
- Milk and sugar are not added to tea in SE Asia, but Tibetan tribes sometimes add salt and yak butter to their tea.
- All teas contain antioxidant polyphenols, but green tea contains more than the others, and is the most popular tea across SE Asia.
- Matcha is made by processing green tea leaves into a green powder, which can be mixed into other liquids or foods.
- L-theanine in tea counterbalances the effect of caffeine, which turns tea into a calming and relaxing beverage.
- Chai tea is a deliciously spiced black tea, made by adding an aromatic spice mix such as ginger, cinnamon, cardamom, vanilla, black pepper, and clove. Best to drink without milk or sugar.
- Ginger root can have a calming effect on an upset stomach and ease inflammation. Ginger in a morning beverage may reduce appetite and increase fullness (Jiang, 2019).

Vegetables

The regions of SE Asia and northern and southern Europe have many vegetables in common, such as mushrooms, potatoes, eggplant, carrots, celery, fennel, radish, and chili. Vegetables in the onion family can give a flavour boost, but upset the stomach, which is why onions and garlic are forbidden in Buddhism.

By far the most prolific, versatile, and nutritious vegetables, with more than 400 known varieties across Europe and Asia, are the brassica family (also called cruciferous):

- leafy green brassicas (cabbage, kale, arugula, cress, bok choy, wombok, mustard greens, choy sum, silverbeet, mizuna),
- fleshy brassicas (broccoli, broccolini, cauliflower, and Brussels sprouts),
- starchy root and stem brassicas (radish, daikon, wasabi, horseradish, rutabaga, swede, turnips, kohlrabi, maca, mashua),
- seed crop brassicas (mustard seed, rapeseed).

Cruciferous vegetables are an excellent source of vitamins C, E, K, calcium, folate, zinc, iron, magnesium, carotenoids (provitamin A), calcium, and fibre. The glucosinolates (which gives cabbage its sulphurous smell) may help slow the growth of cancer cells, and the antioxidant properties of the flavonoids might help reduce systemic inflammation (Caballero, Finglas and Toldra, 2016).

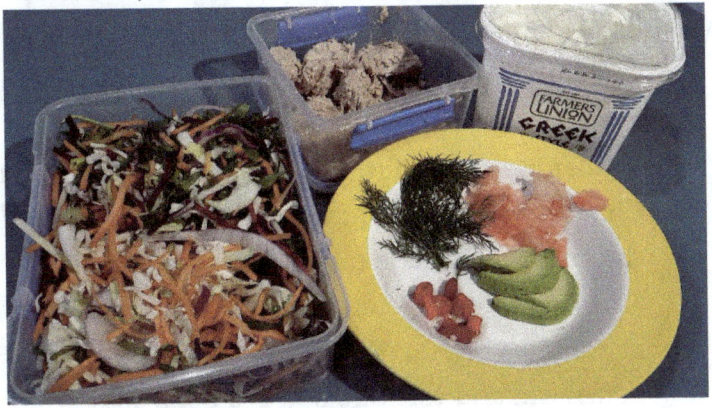

Popular on Italian antipasto plates, the giardiniera salad is a mix of pickled vegetables such as olives, cauliflower, carrots, peppers, celery, and mustard seeds.

The ancient Greeks revered cabbage for its medicinal qualities, and it may be the most versatile vegetable – eaten raw in a coleslaw salad, fermented into sauerkraut in Europe or kimchi in Korea, or wrapped around seasoned rice and other foods before braising.

European sauerkraut and Korean kimchi are made by salting and packing raw cabbage into a container. Vietnamese versions use kohlrabi and bamboo shoots.

- Sauerkraut is popular across northern Europe as an adjunct to help digest sausages and other meat products. If unpasteurised, sauerkraut contains vitamins A, B, C, K, and U, minerals such as iron, potassium, iodine, calcium, magnesium, manganese and sodium, plus trace amounts of phosphorus, chlorine, cobalt, fluorine, silicon, boron, copper, zinc, sulphur, and selenium. Store-bought sauerkraut is often pasteurized to kill all types of bacteria, including the probiotics (Rezac et al., 2018) so check the labels. But even if it is no longer probiotic, the nutrients in the cabbage make it worthy of inclusion in a balanced diet, and the sourness can take the edge off your appetite.
- Similar to sauerkraut, kimchi is a spicy, pungent mix of Chinese cabbage fermented with salt, garlic, ginger, shrimp paste, daikon radish, scallions, red pepper flakes and sugar. Koreans consider it essential to everyday life. It contains vitamins A, B and C as well as iron, potassium and calcium, and is a good source of dietary fibre.

Chapter 7: How did you get so fat?

"How did you get so fat?" my elderly mother asked, with a directness lacking empathy or apology. Dementia, drugs and old age had blunted her memory and sharpened her tongue. I had overcome cancelled flights and volcanic ash clouds to be by her side at the end, but I suddenly felt like an errant child forced to defend myself. How do you answer a question like that?

For years I blamed my family for everything bad that happened to me. It is so much easier to blame others; you can just walk away and leave them far behind; forget they're there, and just get on with your life. But what do you do when you start blaming yourself instead? You can't ignore the voice in your head that keeps telling you it is all your own fault, so you try to drown it out any way you can.

You become an expert at avoidance, developing addictive behaviours as the perfect coping strategies. You engage in excessive bouts of whatever floats your boat – exercise, alcohol, sex, drugs, food, lavish spending sprees, and other self-destructive activities – routinely rebounding off each other like a pinball machine.

But instead of finding peace, your sense of guilt and remorse throws you against the wall and triggers another episode of excess. Strung out like an addict looking for the next fix, you can't think straight. You make more terrible decisions, dig an even deeper hole, and before long you're hitting rock bottom.

It is the stuff of nightmares, and a very lonely place. This is your deep, dark secret. Obesity and depression are partners in your self-destruction. Your mind and body are working against you. Ok, I know that all sounds a little melodramatic, but that is my story.

Most people who write these books have never been grossly overweight. They don't understand, but I do. So, let's face this together and take a long hard look at our relationship with food, from a fat person's perspective, our perspective.

By sharing a few of my own challenges and insights, I hope to prompt a few 'ah ha' moments from you. And when you see your own story reflected in these pages, maybe something will click and it will start to make sense for you too. We need to understand all the reasons why we eat the way we do, so we can stop blaming ourselves and get on with life.

Food-related memories

The hypothalamus is a busy little organ located in the control centre of the brain. Not only does it play a crucial role in telling us WHEN to eat (or stop eating), but it also provides input into WHAT we eat, WHERE we eat, and WHY.

First and foremost, it is an endocrine organ, responsible for sending hormones to wherever they're needed. But it does double shifts in the brain's limbic system too, the region that manages our emotional and behavioural responses.

The limbic system is where we store memories linked to our emotional experiences, and where we form new memories. We store memories in much the same way as a computer stores information. Short-term memories are kept just long enough to complete their immediate purpose, whereas long-term memories are stored, indexed and cross-referenced for future retrieval.

We might forget where we parked the car a few hours ago, but we can somehow remember things from our childhood. Each new long-term memory is linked to one or more existing memories, providing context and an effective cross-reference. Memories can be triggered by sensory cues (sight, sound, smell, taste, touch) and other environmental factors (people, places, events).

When you go to the beach or smell the ocean, you might crave ice-cream or fish-and-chips because you have memories linking them together. A night at the movies might prompt you to want popcorn or chocolates. Christmas celebrations can trigger anticipation for turkey or baked ham with all the trimmings, and birthdays are when you want cake.

Memories can have emotional linkages too. After a tough day you might reach for a drink; when you're feeling sick you might crave chicken soup; or when you're feeling sad you might dial for a pizza. Because so many memories have food associations, the remembering can work both ways. When eating a particular food, it might spark a memory of something else. The sight, touch, taste, or smell of a food can evoke strong memories, some good, some bad.

What food-related memories spring to mind for you? Go to your DIET DIARY and jot them down. I've entered my previous examples into the chart below, as an example of how yours might look. (We'll look at them again later when we start thinking about alternatives.)

Sensory stimulus (memory)	Food related to the memory
Go to beach and smell ocean	Ice-cream, fish-n-chips
Watch movies	Popcorn, chocolate
Xmas	Roast turkey dinner with ham
Birthdays	cake
Tough day at work	alcohol
Sick in bed	Chicken soup

So many of our favourite foods are those we remember from childhood. They remind us how it felt to be children. Not all childhood memories are good ones, so we might like or dislike a food based on whether the attached memories are good or bad. I remember the soothing creaminess of a French vanilla slice from my childhood, so I struggle to walk past them, even now. But I also remember foods I associate with unhappy memories, so I never go near them.

The ability to recognise foods we should eat or avoid is a primitive survival instinct. We automatically seek out the foods with pleasant memories attached. When we eat those foods, our brain conjures up those feelings as a sudden rush of pleasure. Over time, this connection can be 'reinforced' to the point that our conscious mind believes the food itself has the power to make us feel good. If we rely on food in this way, it can lead to EMOTIONAL EATING, where our desire to eat is driven by emotion rather than hunger or nutritional needs, and this can become a major obstacle to weight loss.

Not all memories have links to food, but food-related ones can make us fat. Our food memories are some of our strongest and most powerful; they can engage all our senses, and often have emotional attachment. Not all food memories are pleasant, but they are all triggered by sensory stimulation. The good ones are 'positively reinforced' by a pleasing outcome, and if repeated often enough they quickly become habitual 'learned behaviours' (Epstein et al., 2007). These pleasure-seeking food-related habits are hard to change.

Thankfully we can change existing connections in the brain and make new ones (neuroplasticity). We can retrain our brains to lessen the emotional responses attached to selected memories, and we can create new healthy memories too. But our food behaviours cannot be changed overnight. The old behaviours and responses were reinforced by repetition, over many years, so it will take time to change them.

Eating for pleasure

We've just talked about how our behaviours are linked to our food memories, how those foods give us pleasure, and how these reward-based experiences reinforce our food-seeking behaviours. In other words, certain foods give us pleasure, our mind creates memories linking those foods to feelings of pleasure, so that every time we think of those foods we anticipate a rush of pleasure. This desire for instant gratification can send us foraging in the fridge, the kitchen cupboard, or to desperately dialling the nearest fast-food delivery. Food manufacturers know this. Food retailers know this. And companies that spend a fortune on television advertising know this.

For most of us who are overweight, the most challenging time is often those few hours between dinner and going to bed, when we sit with our eyes glued to the television. The sensory cues can be too much to resist when we see delicious food and smiling faces in every ad break.

Food gives us pleasure. We love it. And the feeling is completely natural. Eating a favourite calorie-dense food like pizza can flood the brain with neurotransmitters called dopamine – the 'feel good' hormones. These hormones attach to the opioid receptors on neurons in the brain, activating intense feelings of pleasure and euphoria (Tuulari et al., 2017). But the pleasurable effect is fleeting, which motivates us to keep eating (Flanagan, 2017).

Our mouth, not our stomach, senses pleasure from the food we eat

Addicts get the same kind of rush from alcohol, tobacco, drugs, gambling, casual sex, or other risk-taking behaviour, but does that make food an addiction too? Maybe. But unlike other addictions, we need to eat multiple times a day. We cannot avoid it, so we must learn to live with it, in moderation, something other addicts are unable to do.

Interestingly, that hit of dopamine that we crave is greater when the food is in our MOUTH, not our stomach. This is especially true when the taste of the food matches our expectations. Ever wondered why your skinny friends always want a spoonful of your dessert? It's because they already know that the joy of eating is in the MOUTH, not the gut (Thanarajah et al., 2019). And this little nugget of truth is powerful. It will set you free.

Appetite and the h unger hormones

Scientists have discovered that adipocytes (fat cells) do much more than simply store excess energy. In fact, they are more metabolically active than previously thought.

They secrete at least six bioactive proteins, two of which, leptin and adiponectin, are nicknamed the 'hunger hormones'. Adiponectin is involved in glucose regulation and the metabolism of fatty acids in protein, whereas leptin has an important role in appetite regulation. But when we have too many fat cells, they release too much leptin and not enough adiponectin, which means that the fatter we become, the more unbalanced this system becomes (Lo, 2018).

With such comparatively low levels of adiponectin in the bloodstream, this can upset the regulation of blood glucose levels and cause cells to become insulin-resistant in a pre-diabetic way. This can make you feel tired, listless, sleepy, and brain fogged.

Because the cells are being starved of glucose, they send urgent messages to the control centre in the brain (the hypothalamus) to send them food, INCREASING APPETITE. But as we keep eating more than we really need, the excess glucose has nowhere to go and starts putting pressure on fat cells for a place to stay.

Overwhelmed by the demand, fat cells send leptin hormones to the hypothalamus in the brain to DECREASE APPETITE and to stop the constant bombardment. But when these conflicting hormonal messages happen too often, the hypothalamus stops responding. It's like getting too much junk mail; eventually you stop reading them and just delete.

But when the hypothalamus stops responding, it's as though a 'hunger switch' in the brain gets stuck in the ON position. Appetite never turns off, we never feel satisfied, we keep eating, and we keep gaining weight. BOOM.

We know that people with normal amounts of body fat have no problem receiving the body's signals to stop eating, but as we gain weight, those signals become weaker, or even non-existent. It has nothing to do with the mythical 'willpower' argument. It is pure biology and neuroscience. The fatter we are, the greater the hormonal imbalance, and the less likely we are to ever feel full, so we keep eating, and we keep getting fatter. It becomes a self-perpetuating cycle of dysfunction.

So how do you reset that hunger switch? You need to lose weight. Ha! Just lose weight, she says. That's all you need do, she says. But even if we do lose weight, the challenges don't stop there. And here is the catch. The body's primitive survival instinct is to store fat for those lean times when food isn't available, so if we start eating a lot less, our body will sense the change and increase our appetite to compensate.

What chance do you have if your own body is fighting you every inch of the way? It can feel like it sometimes. This is one of the reasons our appetite can increase once we do start to lose weight, and why we so often revert to eating too much and regain even more than we lost!

So how do we lose weight and keep it off? We need to lose weight without triggering the body's survival instincts, by eating the right foods in a balanced diet. After only a few short weeks, I felt my natural appetite signals returning, as if the hunger switch had been turned OFF at last. Feeling satisfied after eating is such a blessing after so many years of feeling hungry all the time.

Eating with depression

Depression is not simply a state of low mood, or when you feel anger, fear, sadness, disappointment, or grief. Clinical Depression is a disease state that occurs regularly, making it impossible to function normally, and lasting for hours, days or weeks.

In the grips of a depressive episode, we can experience a 'brain fog'; our thinking becomes vague and sluggish; we feel disconnected from ourselves and everything around us. Nothing seems real. Consequences fail to register. It's like watching someone else open the fridge door, the freezer, the pantry, reaching inside for anything sweet, salty and oily – chips, chocolate, ice-cream, biscuits, pizza, fried food – anything we can get our hands on, so we can 'feel better'.

In the midst of a full-blown episode, we can enter a scary alternate reality where we feel a sense of drowning or suffocating, unable to express happiness or pleasure, and emotionally numb (Berridge and Kringelbach, 2015). This is what some people describe as the 'black hole' of depression.

For a time, we are not our true selves. We transform from the rational Dr Jekyll to his uncontrollable alter-ego Mr Hyde. We can act impulsively, erratically, and without a clear appreciation of consequences. We are prone to irrational thinking, grand gestures, and risky behaviours. At its worst, a type of manic euphoria can take hold. This might last for days or weeks at a time; more than enough time to make some serious mistakes which can have dire consequences.

The extent of the havoc we wreak is largely dependent on the intensity and duration of each depressive episode. But once the fog clears, we become painfully aware of the damage, whether it is fractured relationships, less money in the bank, or extra kilos on the scales.

Sadly, some people don't even need a depressive episode to act this way. Anyone feeling extreme stress or overwhelm can become just as irrational, seeking out short-term pleasure without any thought of long-term consequences. This craving for instant gratification becomes so intense that we cannot envisage any other antidote to our emotional distress. We look for an easy way out, a 'quick fix', and the notion becomes tantalisingly irresistible because it promises an instant dopamine rush, and an end to feeling bad, even if it is short-lived.

We need to break the cycle of depression and binge-eating

Not everyone reaches for food, but we do, don't we? How many times have you been on a diet for a few weeks, lost a few kilos, then undone all that effort with a massive binge session?

Have you struggled with obesity and depression? If so, like me, you may have tried for years to lose weight, but something always happens to derail or undermine your best efforts. You lose motivation and slip back into old habits. Autopilot kicks in and you head for the fridge. It's as if your conscious brain stops working, and your body is hell-bent on harming itself. Any hint of self-control flies out the door and you regress into binge-eating.

People who overeat during a depressive episode are more likely to binge on 'comfort foods' because they promise the greatest level of reward-based pleasure. We tap into food memories to identify the most binge-worthy foods, then we embark on a food marathon. With a fatalistic mindset, we indulge until we feel sick. Only then do we stop. When we realise what we have done, we berate ourselves for being so weak. Our self-esteem and self-worth take another hit, and we panic about gaining more weight!

But what if I told you, it is not all your fault? What if I told you that your gut microbiota made you do it? Yes, that is the latest theory, and there is evidence. The very latest research points to a powerful relationship between mood and food which goes way beyond thoughts of sugar highs, dopamine hits, or satisfying the reward centres of the brain. Food science and neuroscience have found common ground.

Obesity, inflammation, depression

Fat cells secrete pro-inflammatory cytokines (PIC). When we carry too much fat, we release excessive amounts of PIC into the bloodstream,
- stimulating pain centres,

- over-activating the immune response, and
- sending signals to the vagus nerve, which links into the hypothalamic-pituitary-adrenal axis (HPA), influencing our behaviour and triggering depression (Limbana, Khan and Eskander, 2020).

Chronic pain and inflammation increase the risk of developing chronic inflammatory diseases (CIDs) – rheumatoid arthritis, inflammatory bowel disease (IBD), ulcerative colitis, Crohn's Disease, lupus, multiple sclerosis, sinusitis, periodontitis, asthma, tuberculosis, peptic ulcer, heart disease, stroke, cancer, diabetes and Alzheimer's (Zhang and An, 2007; Park et al., 2018).

And life is not fair. If we have one inflammatory disease, we are more likely to develop others; and if we have gut problems we are more likely to suffer mood and cognitive disorders (Limbana, Khan and Eskander, 2020).

The relationship between obesity, inflammation and chronic pain is not new, but the discovery of a link between inflammation and depression adds a new dimension (Franks and Atabaki-Pasdar, 2017).

Include foods with anti-inflammatory properties, such as magnesium, folate, riboflavin, thiamine, zinc, omega-3 fatty acids, and indigestible fibre. Fruit, vegetables, seafood, and wholegrains are excellent food sources, and should be front and centre in any well-balanced diet. To further improve our dietary inflammatory index, we should reduce saturated fats and trans fats, by consuming less fast food, cakes and desserts. (Muhammad et al., 2017).

Obesity as a communication failure

People of normal weight just don't understand how the rest of us can get so fat. They look at us with disdain because they think we simply lack willpower, are lazy, and we eat too much!

"Just put the food down", they say.

"Keep your hand away from your mouth!" they laugh.

They offer no sympathy or empathy, and are blind to the fact that obesity is about so much more than calories and conscious decisions. Yes, we do get fat when we eat more than our body needs, but it is not that simple. Somewhere along the line our relationship with food got all messed up. No matter how much we ate, we never felt full, and the more we ate, the more we wanted.

The gut is supposed to know when we have eaten enough, and it should send signals to the brain to produce a feeling of fullness (satiety), so we know when to stop eating.

The latest obesity research suggests that the reason we keep eating is due to a communication failure between the gut and the brain (Scheja and Heeren, 2019). Messages fail to get through, so we keep eating, and if this happens too often, we gain weight.

In depression, we now know there is a dysregulation in both the neuro-endocrine and neuro-immune communication pathways (Limbana, Khan and Eskander, 2020). And the latest obesity research has found evidence of a two-way communication highway between our gut microbiota (good bacteria living in our gut) and that part of the central nervous system (CNS) that helps modulate behaviours influenced by stress and anxiety (Bliss and Whiteside, 2018).

With the gut and brain working in this bi-directional manner, they could easily affect each other's functions and significantly impact stress, anxiety, depression, and cognition (Carabotti et al., 2015; Limbana, Khan and Eskander, 2020). What this means is that our gut health could directly impact our mental health (and vice versa). This complex array of neural pathways is known as the **gut-brain axis** (GBA) (Cani, 2018).

Role of the Gut-Brain-Axis (GBA)

The systems within the GBA work together to keep us alive:

- The limbic system, which lies within the brain, consists of tiny organs responsible for emotions and memories. The hypothalamus is one of the busiest of these organs, producing hormones to regulate our appetite, mood, temperature, thirst, sleep, and libido.
- The central nervous system (CNS) is the major communication highway linking the neurons of the brain and spinal cord to influence other systems within the body, such as gastro-intestinal system (GIT).
- An estimated 100 million neurons (nerve cells) in the GIT make up the enteric nervous system (ENS), which manages our digestive and intestinal functions. These GIT neurons can produce such an array of neurotransmitters (specialised signalling hormones) that people are calling the gut our 'second brain'.

Our gut can affect our thinking and emotions

Scientists have confirmed that the trillions of resident bacteria in the gut play a major role in the GBA, and using the latest DNA sequencing technologies, they have identified the predominant bacterial species – 90% firmicutes and bacteroidetes, with about 10% actinobacteria (Rinninella et al., 2019). But despite such similarities, every person's gut microbiota may be unique, so we don't yet know what a 'normal' population of gut microbiota is supposed to look like.

What we do know is that people with similar health conditions have remarkably similar gut microbiota – with more of some types of bacteria and less of others (Ju, 2019).

- In obesity and other disease states, large numbers of certain strains of gut bacteria are thought to be interfering with GBA communication via the vagus nerve – causing problems with homeostasis, appetite regulation, and food reward signalling (Alonso et al., 2008).
- Other studies have reported that the types of gut microbiota in the obese could be so different that they alter how the body uses energy and how it converts the excess into fat deposits (Patterson and Sears, 2017).
- Even more recent studies have found that people with depression share the same predominant species of gut bacteria (Limbana, Khan and Eskander, 2020).

It is unclear whether changes in the gut microbiota contribute to the development of these conditions, or if the gut microbiota changes as a secondary consequence of the illnesses. What we do know is that the population and diversity of our gut bacteria is influenced by our DNA, our gut physiology, our use of antibiotics, our health status, our diet and lifestyle, and our external environment. Some of these factors cannot be avoided, but we can try to improve our diet and lifestyle.

Gut hormones respond to the nutrients detected in what we eat, and these food-related responses are thought to initiate most of the communications and signalling between the gut and brain. Evidence suggests that regular consumption of prebiotic foods may assist the GBA by promoting better communication between the gut and the brain.

If we eat enough nutrient-rich food, the gut can signal the brain to reduce appetite. But if most of our food has poor nutrient value, the cells feel starved, so the gut sends signals for us to keep eating. But despite eating lots of calories, we continue to feel lethargic; physically, mentally and emotionally exhausted – an early warning sign that your internal systems are struggling. To prevent or remedy this, we need to eat a BALANCED DIET with FOODS HIGH IN NUTRIENT VALUE, such as fruit, vegetables, seafood, grains, and fermented dairy products.

Prebiotic foods feed our good gut bacteria

Emerging evidence suggests the GBA is somehow involved in the production of its own folate, short-chain fatty acids (SCFAs), and crucial neurotransmitters such as serotonin and gamma amino butyric acid (GABA) (Cani, 2018). If so, this mini ecosystem could influence weight gain in ways we never thought possible – through energy harvesting, SCFA signalling, behaviour modification, appetite control, and modulating inflammatory responses, all of which are implicated in obesity (Frausto et al., 2021).

The gut bacteria are alive, so they need to feed, but the food we eat will determine which species thrive and which will die (Frausto et al., 2021).

- The indigestible fibre in plant food acts as the ideal substrate for microbial fermentation in the gut, resulting in the production of SCFAs – a crucial energy source for healthy gut bacteria.
- Consumption of prebiotic fibres has been shown to activate the central hypothalamic regions of the brain involved in appetite suppression (Kovatcheva-Datchary and Arora, 2013).
- Prebiotic foods containing oligofructose (such as dandelions, bananas, wheat, onions, asparagus, rye and barley) have been linked to improvements in gut nutrient-sensing mechanisms of the GBA, thereby having a positive effect on the endocannabinoid systems that regulate appetite, sleep, memory, pain-sensation, and mood (Bliss and Whiteside, 2018).

Probiotics may help reduce inflammation

An 8-week randomised, double-blind, placebo-controlled clinical trial of 40 patients with diagnosed major depressive disorder (MDD) found that treatment with a probiotic capsule containing three strains of gut bacteria (Lactobacillus acidophilus, Lactobacillus casei, and Bifidobacterium bifidum) reduced inflammation and depression. They concluded that probiotics could reduce the symptoms of depression in the obese, and reasoned that (1) inflammation is implicated in the pathophysiology of depression, and (2) probiotic consumption reduces inflammation (Park et al., 2018).

Studies using probiotic treatment with strains of bacteria known to inhabit the gut (Lactobacilli and Bifidobacterium) reported

- reduced depression in patients with IBD,
- enhanced cognitive reactivity to depressed mood, and improved hypothalamic-pituitary axis response to acute psychological trauma,
- increased fat loss in obese women, with increased satiety, decreased food cravings, lower levels of depression, and improved body image with increased self-esteem, and
- altered concentrations of gut hormones have been linked to improvements in higher brain functions such as sleep, arousal and anxiety (Bliss and Whiteside, 2018).

Scientists are excited by the prospect that dietary manipulation with prebiotics and probiotics could reduce inflammation and oxidative stress in the liver, increase production of gut hormones, control appetite signals, and reduce the growth of fat cells (Kovatcheva-Datchary and Arora, 2013). This is supported by findings of many earlier studies trialling probiotic treatments to address the link between obesity, depression and systemic inflammation (Kovatcheva-Datchary and Arora, 2013).

If probiotic treatment can help alleviate these conditions, then it might be possible to treat the underlying cause instead of the symptoms, challenging the widespread use of anti-inflammatory medications, bariatric surgery, and antidepressants. Only time will tell.

Eat a balanced diet with foods high in nutrient value, such as fruit, vegetables, seafood,

Chapter 8: How much is enough?

How are you feeling at this point? Has reality hit hard? Are you shocked or relieved? Do you feel hopeful of the future? Are you ready to lose weight? How much can you expect to lose? What is a realistic expectation?

When you undergo weight loss surgery or start a new diet, there are no guarantees. Your personal situation is unique. There is no way of knowing what your weight loss will be, what complications you might have, or how much trouble you will have keeping the weight off. Each one of us is different. We face different challenges in our daily lives.

But what I can offer you are the results collected from studying thousands of other people, and from that data we get an indication of what most overweight people can expect to achieve when trying to lose weight.

Any weight loss can improve health

Clinical studies have consistently shown that if an obese person can lose more than 10-15kg they have a good chance of reversing or substantially improving their T2D diagnosis, regardless of which type of diet protocol they use to lose the weight – VLCD, Mediterranean Diet, low-carb diet, or intermittent fasting (Watson, 2018). The following chart shows how relatively small percentages of weight loss can significantly improve major medical conditions (Magkos et al., 2016).

Weight loss %	Clinically significant improvements to medical conditions and risk factors
2-5%	Polycystic ovarian syndrome, infertility
5%	10% reduction in total fat mass, 9% reduction in intra-abdominal fat tissue, 13% intra-hepatic triglyceride; Improved blood pressure, blood glucose, lipid profiles; Improved psychological wellbeing; Reduced plasma concentration of risk factors for cardiometabolic diseases (glucose, insulin, triglycerides, alanine transaminase, leptin); Improved insulin sensitivity in liver and adipose tissue,
5-10%	Reduced overall health care costs
5-16%	Profound improvements in CVD and T2D risks; Continued improvement to muscle insulin sensitivity;
10-15%	Reduced sleep apnea, non-alcoholic fatty liver (NAFL)
11%	18% reduction in total fat mass, 23% reduction in intra-abdominal fat tissue, 52% intra-hepatic triglyceride
16%	27% reduction in total fat mass, 30% reduction in intra-abdominal fat tissue, 65% intra-hepatic triglyceride;
16%+	Reduced plasma concentrations of free fatty acid and CRP inflammatory markers, and increased adiponectin

An obese person can expect profound improvements in their risk profile for cardiovascular disease and diabetes if they can lose between 5-16% of their body weight (Ryan and Yockey, 2017). Even as little as 5% can have a beneficial effect on blood pressure, blood glucose, lipid profiles, and psychological wellbeing. For a person weighing 100kgs, 5% is as little as 5kgs. What an amazing return for minimal time and effort!

And it gets even better. We now know that when you lose fat mass, the fat lodged in and around our liver and other internal organs (the intra-abdominal and intra-hepatic fat) is the first to go. Yay! And as you lose more weight (5-16%), other tissue types begin to benefit. So the more you lose, the healthier you become (Magkos et al., 2016). How exciting is that! What excellent motivation!

Dieticians keep telling us to take it slow and steady, because we can't hope to lose huge amounts of weight overnight and keep it off! But recent studies show evidence in favour of a short, sharp, and intense start to a weight loss diet, making the first few kilos come off quickly. Seeing the immediate weight loss keeps you motivated, and the studies suggest the long-term effects are better for keeping it off. Start strong, then ease out a little, aiming for one kilo a week (Purcell et al., 2014).

But whether you're in the kickstart phase or the long haul, always keep it nutritionally balanced. Don't do anything drastic or it could have serious health consequences. You don't want to lose weight by doing something silly, then get sick and put it all back on again!

Kickstart those first few kilos, but then slow and steady wins the race. If you can consistently lose one kilo a week, that is exactly where you want to be. Ideally, you need to continue new behaviours for at least 3-6 months so they can become normal routine habits for the rest of your life.

Probability of achieving 'normal' weight

According to the BMI calculators, my 'normal weight' would be 60kg, with a BMI of 22. But for me, I know this is unrealistic. I don't remember ever weighing as little as 60kgs, even as a child! But I do remember what it felt like at 70-75kg, and I liked it, so for me this is a realistic 'ideal' weight. However, I know that given my age and physical limitations, I would be thrilled to achieve 85kgs.

When I started this diet, I accepted the realistic goal of 85kgs. It felt achievable, and I made it even easier by breaking it down into mini goals of 10kg increments. I kept telling myself I only had to lose 10kgs, and it only took a few weeks to achieve. Then I set myself another mini goal of 10kgs, and that took only a few weeks. Before long I had lost the first 35kgs, and was so easy. I was so happy.

Once I had lost that 35kgs I was halfway to my goal weight. I was at my primary end point, halfway to my goal. I had lost 50% of my excess weight. This is the same result someone might expect if they underwent weight loss surgery, but following a balanced diet doesn't have any of the associated risks or long-term health issues of surgery.

What does your 'normal weight' look like?
- If you haven't done so already, go to an online BMI calculator of your choice and enter your current weight and height. Write the calculated BMI in your DIET DIARY.
- Then have some fun with the calculator. Enter a few different body weights and watch how the BMI changes

as you lose weight. Keep going until you reach a BMI just below 25. At that point, you would be around 'normal' weight for your height (according to the BMI charts). Take note of the 'normal' BMI and the matching weight, and write it in your DIET DIARY. While considering this suggested weight, decide on a realistic goal weight for yourself, and write it down.

A large longitudinal study (76 704 obese men, 99 791 obese women), with up to 9 years follow-up, found that only a few people managed to reach their 'normal' weight. In the obese group (BMI over 30), the annual probability was only 1 in 210 men and 1 in 124 women. Even fewer in the morbidly obese group (BMI over 40), with only 1 in 1290 men and 1 in 677 women. On a more positive note, the annual probability of achieving a 5% weight reduction was 1 in 8 for men and 1 in 7 for women (Fildes et al., 2015). It helps to have realistic goals.

In a multi-approach trial, a mean weight loss of 5 to 8.5 kg (5-9%) was achieved during the first 6 months, from interventions involving a reduced-calorie diet and/or weight-loss medications, but their weight plateaued at around 6 months. In studies extending to 48 months, a mean 3 to 6 kg (3-6%) of weight loss was maintained. In contrast, those who were only given advice or exercise experienced the least amount of weight loss at any time point (Franz et al., 2007).

Weight loss after surgery

When the NHMRC recommended bariatric surgery in their 2013 clinical guidelines, they lacked follow-up data on the success of weight loss surgery (AIHW, 2017). Hence, the only data we have available is from potentially biased sources. For example, the Bariatric Surgery Registry (BSR), a recent initiative of the Obesity Surgery Society of Australia and New Zealand (OSSANZ), offers a sample of patient follow-up data at 12 months and two years after initial surgery.

The BSR data suggests that the loss of excess weight in the first year after surgery <u>averages</u> at about 50%, with very little change at the 12-month follow-up (Monash University, 2016). Depending on their starting weight, this could be a total loss of only 20, 30 or 40 kgs. If the calculations interest you, here are two practical examples:

Example 1: Female with a BMI of 40 (height 170cm, weight 116kg).
- Based on her height, she would need to weigh only 72kg for a 'normal' BMI of 25.
- The difference between her current weight (116kg) and her target weight (72kg) is 44kg.
- With 44kg of 'excess weight', a 50% loss would equate to 22kg.
- A loss of 22kg would see her weight drop to 94kg (BMI 32.5) not 72kg (BMI 25).
- It's enough to almost get her out of the 'obese' categories but anything over BMI 25 is still considered 'overweight'.

Example 2: Female with a BMI of 48 (height 170cm, weight 145kg).
- Based on her height, she would need to weigh only 72kg for a 'normal' BMI of 25.
- The difference between her current weight (145kg) and her target weight (72kg) is 73kg.

- With 73kg of 'excess weight', a 50% loss would equate to 36.5kg.
- A loss of 36.5kg would see her weight drop to 108.5kg (BMI 37.4) not 72kg (BMI 25).
- She has managed to drop from class 3 'morbidly obese' to class 2 'moderate obese', and no doubt she feels a whole lot better, but her level of risk for obesity-related health conditions remains high.

A substantial weight loss can have a profoundly positive impact on health and wellbeing, but you need to be realistic in your expectations. Most surgical patients can expect to lose HALF of their EXCESS WEIGHT, but most DO NOT reach their 'ideal' weight.

Dieting for weight loss

Can we turn back the clock, even a little? The answer is yes, but we must act smarter, and with intent. We must believe that our lives can improve if we lose a few kilos, not just to improve how we look, but to improve how we feel!

Meta-analyses of clinical studies into the Mediterranean-style and other high-fat diets found that they reduced CVD risk more than low-fat versions. Nuts and full-fat yoghurt were associated with lower rates of weight gain compared to high carbohydrate foods, and high-fat/low-carb diets were best for long-term weight loss (Anton et al., 2017). But be careful. Despite the weight loss, the health benefits and safety of diets with less than 45% carbohydrate (Atkins, Paleo, Keto) have been questioned (Anton et al., 2017).

It might surprise you to know that adults on low-fat/high-carb diets had an increased risk of premature death, they had more trouble maintaining weight loss, and were more likely to gain weight (Ludwig, 2016).

Health issues aside, a large Stanford University study found very little difference between low-fat and low-carb diets for weight loss. Over 12 months, all participants lost between 5-25kg. But most participants lost even less than 5% of their starting body weight, which for someone starting off at 100kg would be less than 5kg (Gardner et al., 2018). That's not much over an entire year of dieting!

A 6-month study of 811 overweight and obese patients measured the effects of calorie-reduced diets with varying amounts of each of the macronutrients (protein, fats, carbs). Average weight loss was 6kg, or about 7% of their starting weight, regardless of which elements were increased or decreased. About 15% of people managed to lose 10% of their starting weight, but that was not the norm (Sacks et al., 2009).

A variety of studies agree that lifestyle interventions involving caloric restriction can typically produce better results, with mean weight losses of 5-10kgs over four to six months (Abete et al., 2010).

Other studies have shown that a combination of calorie restriction (CR) with intermittent fasting (IF) is effective in reducing total body weight (TBW), abdominal fat mass (ABF), and inflammatory markers in overweight or obese patients (Arciero et al., 2016).

Regardless of the type of diet followed, most studies predict that weight loss will plateau after six months, with most people losing only 5-9% of their starting weight (Arciero et al., 2016). Whereas, by creating new behaviours on the HUNGER

HERO DIET, I lost a whopping 24% in 8 months, without exercise, drugs, or surgery. That is a steady and achievable 1kg a week.

> Diets using caloric restriction with intermittent fasting – reduce body weight, abdominal fat, and inflammation

What about exercise?

Don't get me wrong. I have always loved being physical and playing sport; I love the way an exercise session makes me feel. But things change as we age. Old injuries come back to haunt you, limiting what you can do. And life has a way of changing how you live. So, what can we do about it? We need to keep moving.

For our cardiovascular health, we should be aiming for the equivalent of a 20 minute walk every day. A single bout of moderate exercise lasting at least 20 minutes should use up all the glycogen (glucose) stored in the muscles of your arms and legs. By doing this, the liver is forced to release some it its stored energy, the pancreas is kept on its toes producing insulin. This simple 20 minutes a day will help keep the system working and prevent T2D.

If walking for 20 minutes is beyond your current capabilities, don't worry. Just keep this goal in mind for later when you start losing weight and regain mobility.

After losing the first 10kgs, I started to walk more easily around the house and garden, but it took a while longer before

I could progress to a walk around the block or up the street. It can take time, but when it happens you will feel like a million dollars! You will feel younger and more alive. Believe me, it is totally worth it.

Daily stretches help to maintain a functional range of movement... move it or lose it

In the meantime, try to keep using your muscles and joints as much as you can. Do stretches while sitting in a chair, or even while lying in bed. Try to keep your body parts lubricated and moving, or you will start feeling pain in places you didn't know existed.

I try to exercise in a swimming pool every second day or so, paddling slowly back and forth, just to keep my arthritis under control and my lungs working properly. Non-weight-bearing exercises done in the water are excellent therapy for body, mind, and spirit. It is amazing how good you can feel after just a little light exercise. But for now, whatever your circumstances, just aim to keep moving, even if you are sitting in a chair most of the day.

Physical activity is necessary to keep our bodies functioning properly, but don't expect to lose weight if you exercise. In 2012, a group of international scientists from multiple health disciplines published the results of a review they undertook of all major research trials where exercise was used as a weight loss tool. And their findings make it official: **"Regular exercise by itself results in modest loss, or even weight gain"** (Thomas et al., 2012).

Contrary to popular thinking, instead of helping us to lose fat, our bodies respond to exercise by lowering our metabolism to conserve energy. When we exercise to lose weight, a failsafe mechanism called 'metabolic adaptation' lowers our 'resting metabolic rate', conserves energy, increases appetite, and can start breaking down muscle tissue instead of fat. The bathroom scales might show a drop in weight, but you might be losing more muscle than fat.

So don't beat yourself up for not exercising, and don't put unnecessary stressors on your body if you are seriously overweight. Once you lose a few kilos, your body will start to move more easily and you will naturally increase your daily activity. Much later, down the track, you could talk to a health professional about a suitable form of regular exercise or weight training to build strength and conditioning.

Can we keep it off?

I tried for so many years to lose weight, but it always came back, as if my body was fighting me. And I was right. I was not imagining it.

When the body's control systems register a weight loss, they see it as a problem that needs fixing. And we now know that the gut-brain-axis (GBA) is responsible for sending those signals to increase appetite and regain the weight.

So how do we lose weight without triggering a rebound increase in appetite? How do we do it? We trick the sensors by maintaining a nutritionally balanced diet while losing weight, and afterwards. If we avoid nutritional deficits, the weight loss will not trigger any alarms. Interestingly, a balanced diet including full-fat Greek-style yoghurt has been associated with less rebound weight gain.

According to longitudinal survey data, only 1 in 6 overweight or obese adults can maintain their 10% weight loss for more than a year (Ebbeling et al., 2012). Most start to regain weight after only 6 months. However, there is hope.

A systematic review of the literature identified a number of strategies commonly used by those who were the most successful at keeping the weight off – those who could sustain a weight loss of more than 15kg for more than a year (Lowinger, 2015). During both the weight loss and maintenance phases, these successful people:

- Monitor their food intake,
- Monitor their weight,
- Maintain a portion-controlled diet with limited variation,
- Reduce the time spent watching TV, and
- Engage in some form of physical activity every day.

Chapter 9: Are you ready for change?

There are four major risk factors for becoming overweight or obese:
1. Diet – what you eat,
2. Thoughts, beliefs, and behaviours – how you think,
3. Lifestyle – how and where you live, and
4. Nature and nurture elements – genetics and upbringing (Bliss and Whiteside, 2018).

Many people say it's a waste of time trying to change, because obesity runs in their family. They cite 'genetic predisposition' as an excuse to do nothing.

Some will try eating differently, copying some current trend their friends are following, or getting other people to do the shopping and cooking for them. But the novelty soon wears off and they go back to their old ways.

Others will get a burst of enthusiasm from a New Year's resolution, joining a gym, buying a piece of exercise equipment from a TV advertisement, or buying new walking shoes. But the interest wains after a few short days or weeks, and nothing changes.

Then we have a few brave folk who take responsibility for their current situation. It can be confronting, and even distressing, but they face their personal demons, and challenge their long-held beliefs. These people strive to understand themselves, their motivations, and their weaknesses. These people are open to change.

But other people telling us to change can have the opposite effect, making us resist change even more.

Just being aware of the health risks is never enough. Medical research confirms that most of us start taking the information seriously when it finally hits home – as a personal diagnosis, or something happens to someone we care about. But it takes time for the shock and disbelief to shift from contemplation to taking positive action.

Clearly, there are some things we cannot change. We can't go back in history and create a different life, but we do have the power to change how we think and behave.

The older we get, the more set in our ways we become. Our routine behaviours are comfortable and enjoyable, so we resist attempts to change them. We look forward to our morning coffee, our weekend breakfast of bacon, eggs, toast, and all the trimmings. We like the occasional pizza, hamburger, or fish and chips. We like to go out with friends to local restaurants and cafes, to birthday parties and other events. We relax with a glass or two of wine every night, or maybe a scotch. And we like to sit down at night with our feet up and watch TV.

Ok, I'm just guessing here, but you know what I'm saying. Over the years, we develop habits that we enjoy, so we will naturally try to resist having to change them or do without our little treats. But if you refuse to face facts and make some permanent changes, nothing will happen. You will stay the way you are – fat and miserable. I know this from personal experience. Use this chapter as a guide to help you make those changes.

Stages of Change

The most widely acclaimed research into 'behaviour change' in humans has come from decades of clinical studies on how to quit smoking. They found it was difficult to quit, that most would try multiple times before finally giving up for good, and that failed attempts were not about a lack of willpower, but a lack of preparation.

These pioneering researchers concluded that, to successfully change their behaviours, a person must progress through a series of stages, so they called it the Stages of Change (Prochaska, Norcross and DiClemente, 1994). Despite coming from addiction studies, the general principles have been successfully applied to all manner of things we want to change, including our food-related behaviours.

As I became familiar with these stages, something clicked in my head. It all seemed so clear to me, and I realised where I had gone wrong in the past. And something we should all realise is that it might take multiple tries before we get it right. Rome wasn't built in a day, and we should be prepared for a few false starts. That's okay. Pick yourself up, brush yourself off, and think about what you can do better next time. Eventually, it will stick. Planning and persistence are the keys to success.

Stage 1: Pre-contemplation

This is the period of blissful ignorance, when we haven't started thinking about the habits we need to change.

Stage 2: Contemplation

This stage starts when we become aware of a problem. We might look in the mirror, get on the scales, or try on clothes. Or it could be a medical warning for ourselves or others we care about. We start thinking about what we can do to fix the problem. We ask questions and investigate options, seeking advice. We might undergo tests, or spend money on other health services. We might try a fad diet, or other pills and potions. We might even join a gym, but don't go often enough to make a difference. We can spend a lot of time, money, and effort at this stage, without achieving anything. Many people struggle to move past this point. They get stuck here because they think this is all it takes. If they don't know how to move on to the next stage, they feel they have failed – and they keep repeating the same mistakes every time.

Stage 3: Preparation

But some people experience a moment of clarity and conviction. They take personal responsibility for their actions, identify what they need to do, set realistic and achievable goals, and they enter the preparation stage. It is here that we identify potential challenges (physical, emotional, mental, logistical, financial) and decide what we can do to overcome them. With this plan in place, we can soon move forward into the action stage.

Stage 4: Action

In the action stage, you START making those changes you need to make. You START making the right choices and eating the right food. And this is where you must START being a little selfish. Your commitment to your own wellbeing must not be derailed by your sense of responsibility for others. For many, this is the most difficult lesson to learn. But you are worth it. Things must change.

This is where you START using your DIET DIARY every day, writing about your challenges and keeping track of your progress. The action stage is where you make firm commitments to yourself, and begin to follow through with your plan.

Stage 5: Maintenance

Neuroscientists know it can take 6 months for daily routine behaviours to become habits, so once you reach 6 months, you are on the right track for maintaining all those changes. You may not have reached your goal weight by then, but you are well on the way. You have successfully created permanent changes to your behaviours and have substantially reduced the risk of regaining that lost weight.

Which stage are you at right now?

1	Pre-contemplation	I have *never thought* about changing habits
2	Contemplation	I am *thinking* about changing habits
3	Preparation	I have *started* preparing to change habits
4	Action	I have *made* the changes, and doing things differently
5	Maintenance	I have *maintained* the changes for at least 6 months

By reading this book, you have reached at least stage 2 and are contemplating the need to change some things in your life. Or you may have already progressed to stage 3 and are now planning how to make those changes. But the process of change seldom continues in such a linear fashion. You may stall at stage 3 and not move up to take action at stage 4. Or you might lose motivation and slip back to stage 2 where every now and then you might think about what you need to do. Don't feel bad if you slip backwards a few times.

Regression can occur at any stage, so think of it like you're trying to walk up a mountain path with loose stones underfoot. You might lose your footing and slip a few metres down the slope, but once you recover from the fall, you start back up the slope. It's the same when you start progressing through the stages of change. Life has a way of undermining our best intentions. So don't beat yourself up if you slip back to an earlier stage.

Don't expect to be perfect. You are human. But the lesson is not to give up on yourself. It might take a few attempts, but when you are ready to try again, just do it. Believe in yourself. You are worth it.

Setting goals

This goal-setting exercise will help you express your dreams and ground your expectations. Think about the WHAT, WHY, WHEN and HOW. Write notes in your DIET DIARY as you read this chapter, and by the end you should have a much better idea of what your personal goals look like.

What do I want?

Focus on what it is you want to achieve. Be specific. It will not work if all you say is: "I want to lose weight". If you lack a clear direction, you run the risk of losing interest or becoming unmotivated. Being specific about your goals helps you to focus on exactly what it is you want to achieve.

We have talked about how much weight most people can expect to lose. Now it is your turn to decide how much weight YOU want to lose. Do you want to lose 10kg? 20kg? 30kg? More??? Be honest. Be specific. It is okay to aim high, but try to be realistic too. If you are currently more than 40kg above your 'ideal' weight, you might find that losing 20 or 30 kilos is a more realistic goal. Your goals should be challenging; they shouldn't be too easy; but they need to be achievable or else you risk losing hope and giving up.

What is my motivation?

Do you have any OTHER GOALS? Write them down too. Are they connected to your primary goal of losing weight? My secondary goals were about things I knew would improve once I lost weight; like fitting into a favourite pair of jeans, being able to walk along the beach again, or going out with friends. They became my distance markers along the path to my goal weight, showing me how far I had come. For me, they became my motivation.

This is about being honest with yourself, and ensuring what you are trying to achieve is truly worthwhile to YOU. If losing weight is a serious priority for you, this will help you answer the WHY. What is your motivation? What does weight loss mean to you?

Think about your own personal reasons for wanting to lose weight. Be honest. Dig deep. What is your true motivation? In your DIET DIARY, list and describe each reason. E.g.
- I want to lose weight… to feel better about myself.
- I want to lose weight… to fit into my favourite clothes.
- I want to lose weight… to get out and socialise more.
- I want to lose weight… to go for a walk without pain.
- I want to lose weight… because I've had a health scare.

WHAT do I really really want, and WHY?

Now put it all together. Write a **MISSION STATEMENT** that describes your intentions. My own statement might have looked something like this: "I need to lose 35kg so I can stop using a walking stick and fit into my favourite clothes again." With my end goal clearly articulated, I knew exactly what success would look like.

How long will it take?

Every goal needs a target date or else you can flop around forever and go nowhere. A target date will motivate you to apply the focus and discipline needed to do your best to achieve your goals. This answers the WHEN. Set a target date.
- Place a timeframe on reaching your goal weight, which could be as little as 3, 6, or 12 months. For example, at one kilo a week, a weight loss of 40kgs could realistically take 40 weeks.
- Then set yourself mini goals for reaching milestones along the way, e.g., aim for mini goals of 10kgs in 10 weeks.

These mini goals and timeframes are not out in the distance, but so close you can almost touch them. For example,

I estimated it could take more than a year to reach my goal weight, and that filled me with dread. To make it easier – mentally and emotionally – I set mini goals of 10kg. I felt more comfortable thinking about losing 10kg in 3 months; it felt like something achievable, that I could commit to doing.

When I reached that first 10kg weight loss point after only 10 weeks, I was ecstatic. I realised, "I can do this", so I immediately set another mini goal for the next 10kgs. I continued doing this until I reached a weight loss of 35kgs in 8 months.

It sounds like such a simple thing to do, setting mini goals, but you increase your chance of success if you set small achievable goals along the way. And remember, nothing is locked in concrete. You can reassess your goals along the way, and make decisions based on your own progress and circumstances.

Your unique experiences will inform you as you go along. As you navigate your own way through this weight loss experience, you will learn so much more about yourself. You will become the expert on YOU. Embrace the learning experience.

Each of us has the power to change our destiny and live a longer, happier, and healthier life, but we need to let go of all the excuses. Yes, I know you have valid reasons for your current predicament, as we all do, but you need to let them go!

Don't allow limitations to define who you are. You can improve your situation. Free yourself from the mindset of denial. Face the truth. Admit that whatever you've been doing is not working for you. Open your mind to the possibility of a better life. Unlock the chains that have been holding you back. You can do this.

Create SMART mini goals along the way...
make them Specific, Measurable, Achievable,
Relevant, and Timely

Chapter 10: Strive to become your best self

What motivates us? Are we driven by a desire to please others, or is it a more basic human instinct that pushes us to strive for something better?

If we're struggling to pay the bills, or living in a dangerous environment, we can think of little else. Our basic survival takes up every waking moment, and we make decisions based on immediate need rather than long-term wellbeing.

Maslow's famous 1943 paper entitled "A Theory of Human Motivation" explains how we strive to better ourselves. Beyond basic survival needs, humans instinctively strive to be happy. Happiness can mean different things to different people, but a sense of belonging is key to achieving personal growth. With healthy relationships and a strong sense of self, we can become the very best version of ourselves. Maslow called it the 'hierarchy of needs' which is usually represented as sequential levels or steps, set within a pyramid shape (Maslow, 1943).

Basic survival needs are on the bottom level, and we progress upward, one level at a time, toward the pinnacle of self-actualisation where we can become the best version of ourselves. Maslow theorised that once our physical needs are being met, we feel safe enough to start focussing on needs beyond those of basic survival. We branch out beyond ourselves, connecting with others, and building relationships. This marks a turning point. We start believing we are worth it, that life can get better, and our dreams are within reach.

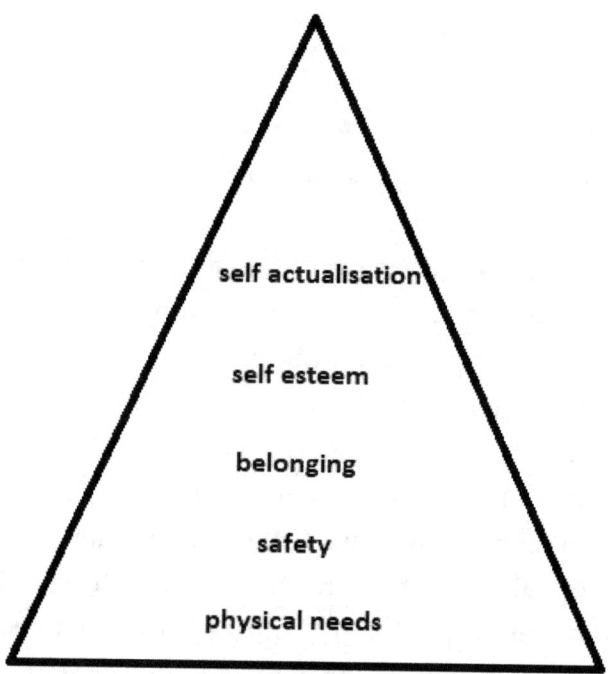

Figure 1: Maslow's hierarchy of needs

1. **Physical needs:** we start here, securing what we need for our basic survival – air, water, food, sleep, and freedom from disease.

2. **Safety**: Once we have our basic survival needs secured, we can feel safe enough to strive for more, moving up the pyramid.
3. **Belonging:** We satisfy a need to belong to a tribe, building strong connections with others who help and support each other.
4. **Self-esteem**: With the support of others, we begin to feel good about ourselves. We have a stronger sense of self-worth, and believe that our dreams are achievable.
5. **Self-actualisation:** This is the pinnacle of personal development; a state of being where we become the best version of our true selves.

Preparing for life's challenges

We all face challenges and obstructions, derailing the best of intentions. Real life is seldom straightforward. We scramble up Maslow's pyramid, meet an obstacle and slide backwards, forced to re-focus on lower-level issues again.

This can happen time and again, just as we start to see real progress, but humans are resilient creatures. We don't give up easily. If our self-esteem is strong, we can pick ourselves up, assess the damage, and try again. We can see misfortune as a momentary setback, not a total ruination of our dreams.

But not everyone can bounce back straight away. We can get stuck in the mire of negative emotions.

The sense of loss can be overwhelming when faced with a relationship breakdown, death of a loved one, being ill, or losing a job. Our brain's coping mechanism starts with denial, then anger. But when we start looking for someone to blame, and lash out, we can hurt ourselves even more. Convinced the world is against us, we find ways to drown our sorrows or get a quick dopamine high. It might be alcohol, drugs, sex, food, excessive physical activity, risky adventures, or lavish spending sprees.

Those who appear resilient can falter too, when faced with similar challenges, but their mindset is a bit different. While the easily overwhelmed person indulges to achieve a short-term escape from their problems, the seemingly more resilient exhibit more bravado than good sense. They choose behaviours that tempt Fate, to prove they are impervious and in control. They see this as the ultimate form of self-determination, however misguided.

Both types of people exhibit extremes of behaviour, and neither is healthy. To stop this from happening over and over, we need to look at why we act the way we do, to break the cycle of self-destruction.

Conditioned responses

Anyone who has trained a pet with food rewards will appreciate how being rewarded for an action has a positive effect on behaviour – and humans are no different.

Any kind of reward makes us feel good, so we look forward to the next opportunity to be rewarded again. Even if the pleasure is fleeting, we are more likely to engage in that behaviour again. We become conditioned to behave in the way that produces a good feeling, and this is called positive reinforcement.

Most of us who are very fat or obese have become conditioned to use food as a coping strategy for when things go wrong. The more times we use food in this way, the more reinforced those food-seeking behaviours become. We might not even realise we are using food in this way, because regular conditioning makes those responses automatic.

The psychology experiments with Pavlov's dog more than 100 years ago showed how we become conditioned. He conditioned his dog to associate the sound of a bell with food. Over time, the dog would anticipate being fed and start salivating, whenever he heard the bell.

Humans are much the same. We become conditioned to associate food with all sorts of things – people, events, smells, memories, etc – but stress is the biggest trigger for most of us. We faced with any of these associations, we literally begin to salivate. There is nothing wrong with this, if we can practice moderation, but most of us struggle with the concept. We always end up eating too much.

Stress can be our undoing. If we're having a bad day, we naturally want to feel better. We know from our past experiences (conditioning) that certain things will give us pleasure, so we go in search of them. But the pleasure is always short-lived. The realisation of what we've done creates more stress, triggering another bout of indulgence to smother the self-loathing – and the cycle continues.

Going back to Maslow's pyramid, we will not reach the top level of self-actualisation if our self-esteem is constantly being undermined by self-loathing.

It took years to become conditioned to using food and other addictions as a way of coping with life, so it will take time to break that conditioning. But you don't do that by getting angry or by blaming yourself for a lack of willpower. That's just the sort of abuse that gets flung at fat people by those who don't understand. It has nothing to do with willpower. It is aboutlearning new ways to react, that don't include food rewards.

Become aware of your triggers. Recognise the things that make you feel bad, the external stimuli that trigger your conditioned response to use food as a 'feel good' reward. In behavioural studies, we use the ABV Method: Antecedent, Behaviour, and Consequence. The antecedent is what triggers the behaviour, and the consequence is how that behaviour makes you feel afterwards (Watson and Tharp, 2007).

Antecedent (stimulus)	Behaviour (reaction)	Consequence (outcome)
Argument with someone. I feel agitated	I eat a chocolate bar and packet of chips	I feel better, but not for long
I feel angry for eating too much	I promise to starve myself for the day, but end up eating even more	I feel worse
It's December, so all the special xmas foods in the shops look so delicious and inviting	I buy chocolate, cakes and fudge. I think I deserve a treat, but I eat them all before xmas day.	Delicious, but I feel bad. Eaten too much and gained weight. Not able to enjoy xmas now.

For example, if you have an argument with someone and feel agitated, what do you do? Maybe you grab a chocolate bar and a packet of chips. You feel better for a few minutes, but then you feel angry at yourself for having no self-control and eating all those extra calories.

To teach yourself a lesson, you promise to starve yourself for the rest of the day. But that only triggers another eating binge, and you feel worse. The following table is how this would look, using the ABC method. (Notice how the outcome on one line can become the trigger of another line. This is the cyclical nature of conditioned responses.)

For at least a week, keep a record in your DIET DIARY of things that prompt you to go looking for food. Include sensory stimuli if you wish, such as seeing ads on TV, but in this exercise, we are most interested in those emotional triggers that are specific to YOU. If you do this simple exercise, you will discover WHAT you are doing, and WHY.

1. **Open** your **DIET DIARY** and create a fresh chart with columns, as you can see in the example.
2. **List** any triggers you already know about, then keep adding to the list over the next week or so until you have at least 6 or more triggers in the first column on your chart.
3. As you list each trigger, fill in the next column with a description of how you reacted.
4. After listing your reaction, consider how you felt afterwards. Write this down in the 'consequence' column.
5. You now have a list of what NOT to do. Can you see a pattern?

Alternate responses

Looking at that previous example, you can see how those food-related behaviours result in poor outcomes. It's not rocket science; we already know it's a problem. And trying to 'teach yourself a lesson' by starving yourself the next day will not have a better outcome! It will not encourage a change of behaviours. It will make you push back and resist the punishment, triggering another binge.

Antecedent (stimulus)	Behaviour (reaction)	Consequence (outcome)
Argument with someone. I feel agitated	My first thought is for a chocolate bar and packet of chips, but I have cheese and crackers instead	Eating always helps me calm down, but this time I made a healthier choice. I feel good about that.
I feel angry for eating too much	I always eat when I'm agitated, but I want to change that reaction. I find a guided meditation on the internet and start practicing.	I managed to calm down without using food. I feel good about myself. This is something I can do.
It's December, so all the special xmas foods in the shops look so delicious and inviting	I wait until later in the month before buying treats, so I can have them for sharing on xmas day.	I feel in control for once. I'm looking forward to xmas now.

The only effective way to create long-term change is by positive reinforcement – choosing to react differently to those triggers, and feeling good about yourself afterwards.

Working with the previous example, I've thought long and hard to come up with some better behaviours, which result in better outcomes. Using the alternate behaviours, I feel better about myself and less likely to binge as a rebound consequence.

Now it's your turn. Using your own examples, find alternative ways you could respond to your triggers. Try to come up with better ways of reacting, which will make you feel good afterwards, and not push you toward a food-related reward.

Find alternate responses that work for YOU. If you sit quietly and consider your options, I think you'll come up with some great ideas.

1. Go to your **DIET DIARY** and create another chart. Use the same column headings as the last one: Antecedent, Behaviour, Consequence.
2. Copy everything from the Antecedent column of the previous chart into the first column of this new chart. Leave the other columns blank.
3. Now take some time to think about how you might have acted differently to each stimulus. Write those ALTERNATE RESPONSES in the Behaviour column.
4. Now think about how you might feel after using the alternate response instead of your usual food-related coping strategy. You should feel better about yourself. If not, go back and re-assess the alternate behaviour and try to think of another option. When you end up with a more positive outcome, write those feelings in the Consequence column of this chart.

Compare both charts. Do you see how the ALTERNATE RESPONSES produce a better outcome? Next time something triggers you, try using an alternate response to food. If you try this often enough, you will start to break all that unhealthy conditioning, and you will feel better about yourself. Life is full of challenges, and the only thing we can hope to control is how we react to those challenges.

Reflect on this and try to think of all the potential barriers to your reaching your goals. Are you prepared to make the necessary changes? What are you prepared to give up to achieve those goals? Be prepared. Look at ways to deal with challenges before they arise, and give yourself a better chance of success. "Will that cake, pie, ice cream, drink, burger, pizza, chips, chocolate, etc, make me happy?"   NO

Others may try to stop you

Human nature can be fickle. Family, friends, acquaintances, and work colleagues may feel threatened when they realise you are trying to lose weight. So don't tell anyone. Keep it to yourself. Don't make a big deal about it. If tempted to tell, just remember Brad Pitt's classic line: "The first rule of Fight Club is: Do NOT talk about Fight Club."

Sure, you need to say something to those you live with before you start clearing the pantry and fridge of temptations, but keep it low key. If you must tell them something, tell them you need to improve your health (which is the truth). Most people will support you if medical issues are involved, but you will find a lot more resistance if you tell them you are planning to lose weight!

Dieting is something everyone seems to have an opinion about, and even strangers are all too willing to tell you what they think. I find it quite disturbing that people you barely know can feel it's quite acceptable to comment on your weight, and repeat all sorts of nonsense they read somewhere on the internet as if they know more than you do. They will even argue the point, just to prove to you how much they think they know. But don't be swayed by these people. If you're successful, it will make them look bad. They don't want you to succeed.

People feel threatened by change, and many will feel afraid they will lose you if you lose weight. This is especially true of intimate partners and close friends – the people closest to you who most likely share the same unhealthy relationship with food as you do. Will they lose their partner in crime – someone who's always up for a session at the pub, a kebab on the way home, or a late-night pizza? Who will they call next time they have a relationship meltdown and need someone to share their angst over a chocolate binge? Who will share in their late-night drink-n-dial tears while tucking into a tub of ice-cream? "Misery loves company", and this can be painfully true.

I know you want to share your hopes and dreams with those around you, but most will try to stop you from changing. "You're not fat", they'll say with a tight smile, trying to undermine your resolve.

Be your own best friend, and trust in yourself

At the start, you will be your most vulnerable and easily swayed to give up, but don't let them get inside your head. Trust yourself. You have looked at the facts, come to a logical conclusion, and made the tough decision to change your relationship with food. This may force changes to your relationships with people too, but that is their problem, not yours. Don't let their fears stop you from living your best life.

Hopefully, once they see you losing weight and feeling happier about yourself, they will come onboard and give you positive encouragement. They may even ask for your secret and follow your example. But remember, you cannot control how others think or act; you can only control your own thoughts and actions.

Kuchisabishii - feed your lonely mouth

Most of what we know about 'behaviour change' has come out of decades of human experimentation into smoking cessation (Prochaska, Norcross and DiClemente, 1994), but the Japanese have a simpler approach. They call it **KUCHISABISHII** – which loosely translates to 'satisfying your lonely mouth'.

The act of smoking or eating is often done mindlessly. The hand-to-mouth action becomes so automatic that we can eat, drink, or smoke without thinking about it. We can develop a habit of opening the fridge door 'just to have a look', every time we walk past the kitchen. We can sit in front of the television and mindlessly stuff snacks into our mouths. According to KUCHISABISHII, we are eating to appease our 'lonely mouth'. Think about that for a second. It sounds weird, but it also makes sense.

A 'lonely' mouth cries out for something to go into it – food, drink, or a cigarette. No surprise we stick a rubber dummy into the mouth of a crying baby, something Freud would have something to say about. But that instinct to pacify a lonely mouth can cause us to eat too much, drink too much, and maybe even smoke too much. People who are constantly grazing or looking for food have a very 'lonely' mouth. The mouth takes over, ignoring messages from the gut and brain to stop searching for food. In effect, the tail is wagging the dog!

Do you suffer from a 'lonely' mouth? Is KUCHISABISHII your worst enemy? If so, don't feel bad. That desire to put something in your mouth is perhaps the strongest natural survival instinct we have, so we cannot expect to control it. But we can try to understand it, and learn to manage it.

Your mouth will always tell you what it wants, so you need to satisfy it or it will keep crying out to be fed. But what does it want? You need to focus on your mouth and listen to it.

Think about your favourite foods. Why do you find them satisfying? Why do they make your mouth happy?

It can be a combination of appearance, smell, texture, and flavour. When the food hits the sensors in our mouth, our mouth will know if it's crunchy, soft, creamy, sweet, sour, bitter, juicy, or umami.

And let's not forget the memories and emotions we attach to certain foods. Foods can make us feel happy, sad, guilty, pleased, satisfied, refreshed, or even more hungry.

- In your **DIET DIARY**, make a list of all your FAVOURITE food and drinks. Be specific. Don't just say 'chocolate' if your favourite brand has a caramel centre. If pizza is your thing, describe your favourite. What about drinks? What are your favourites?
- Now ask yourself WHY you like each of these foods. Is it the TEXTURE – crunchy, or smooth and creamy? Is it the FLAVOUR – sweet, spicy, or a little sour? Is it the SMELL – does it make you salivate in anticipation? And what about the APPEARANCE – does it look fresh and juicy, or hot and sticky?
- In your **DIARY**, beside each food, describe what you like about it. Is it how it looks, smells, tastes, or feels in your mouth? Is it sweet, salty, crunchy, smooth, sour, or umami? Are these foods linked to fond memories? When your mouth is feeling lonely, what makes you look for these foods?

- Now think about alternatives. If you can't think of any, don't worry. In following chapters, we introduce the idea of SMART SNACKS. We give you a few suggestions that are known to work, then you can add your own ideas to the list as you go along.

Use the strategies

We never know what challenges lie ahead, but we can have strategies up our sleeves for when negative thoughts reawaken our 'monkey mind'. Erratic thoughts trigger unhealthy behaviours.

Psychotherapists specialising in behaviour change often use this list of processes to help clients get back on track. You can use them too. Think of them as steps in the Change process – from becoming more self-aware, to learning new behaviours, to seeing how we interact with our external environment.

Use the following list as a reminder of the skills you now possess, and as a prompt when times get tough (Prochaska and Norcross, 2003). You can do this.

Processes of Change	Description
Consciousness-raising	You become more aware and informed about yourself and your problems
Emotional arousal	Experiencing and expressing feelings about one's problems and solutions
Self re-evaluation	The self is re-evaluated with respect to the antecedents and potential solutions to your problems
Self-liberation	The potential for a desirable outcome and the changes required for it are examined in terms of ability and commitment.
Counter-conditioning	Substituting alternatives for problem behaviours
Stimulus control	Avoiding stimuli that trigger problem behaviours
Reinforcement	Rewarding self, or being rewarded by others, for making changes and meeting goals
Helping relationships	Enlisting the help of people who care and being open with them
Environmental re-evaluation	Consider how our problems and their potential solutions may influence our physical environment
Acknowledging affect	Experiencing and expressing how potential solutions will affect your problems

Chapter 11: Self-care for mind and body

Feeling fat and miserable can become a bad habit. We get caught up in thoughts of what we can no longer do, and forget who we really are.

Sometimes we need to remind ourselves of who we are, and tangible evidence of our accomplishments can boost our self-confidence.

If you have any awards or certificates tucked away in boxes, get them out on display. Have them there in front of you, as testament to your achievements. Travel photos are good too, as they trigger memories of exciting times when we knew how to have fun.

To help you remember, we have offered you a few simple exercises to get your brain ticking over. Hopefully they will trigger positive memories, and over time, they will help strengthen your confidence and rebuild your self-esteem.

On a fresh page in your **DIET DIARY**, finish these sentences:

- "I have many personal achievements and successes..." (List at least 20, even if it's learning to cook, drive a car, or having kids.)
- "I can do all of these things really well..." (List at least 20 – maybe you're a great cook, or a good listener.)
- "I have many unique and exceptional qualities..." (List 10. Maybe your special gift is always having time to listen when friends need you.)
- "I think this part of my body is a particularly attractive feature..." (We all have some part of us that we like, so write down at least one.)

Now try reading your answers out aloud, and repeat every morning for a week. Get reacquainted with who you are. Find your inner strength and face each day with head held high. Tell yourself, "I can do this!"

Dry scrubbing

I love the feeling after a relaxing massage, so a few years ago, I treated myself to a day spa, with all the trimmings – dry scrub, mud pack, body wrap, shower spritz, and an aromatherapy massage.

I thought the dry scrub was a bit weird at first, but it's supposed to assist exfoliation and lymphatic drainage – or according to the therapist, it will lift old skin cells and leave me feeling all shiny and new. She was right, and I liked how my skin began to tingle as the blood flow increased beneath the skin.

I remembered this experience when I lost the first 10kgs on the HUNGER HERO DIET. My skin had started to itch and it felt like it needed a good scrub, to get rid of dead skin cells, oils and all the toxins leaving my body as I lost weight. But I couldn't reach my back properly.

I went shopping for a back scrubber but they were expensive. Then I had a brainwave. In the household cleaning aisle of the supermarket, I found a long-handled brush for just a couple of dollars. Ok, it was sold as a toilet brush, but I didn't care. It was a brand-new brush, so it didn't matter that I was going to use it on my skin.

It was a huge success. The long handle made it easy to use, and the nylon bristles gave just the right amount of scrub. I sat naked on the bed and gently scrubbed my back, arms, bottom, and legs. For the delicate skin on my face and chest I used a cosmetic facial cleanser and washed it off in the shower. I did indeed feel all shiny and new.

Calming effect of essential oils

Authentic 'essential oils' are pure undiluted extracts from a variety of leaves, flowers, barks, rhizomes, seeds, and fruit peels of aromatic plants. In folk medicine of many countries, essential oils are credited with antibacterial, anti-inflammatory, analgesic, mood-adjusting, and insomnia-alleviating effects (Zhang and Yao, 2019).

Most of us are familiar with the scent of lemon, lavender, or eucalyptus in our household cleaning agents, but these tend to be artificial chemical copies of the real thing. The 'essential oils' sold cheaply at weekend markets are not true essential oils either.

Pure essential oils can be expensive for a tiny bottle, but you only use a couple of drops at a time. Some of the more common essential oils are available in supermarkets (eucalyptus and tea tree oils), pharmacies, and specialty retail shops (lavender, jasmine, or bergamot). For anything a little more unusual, you need to go online to find a supplier.

My favourite essential oil is **CLARY SAGE**, which is difficult to find in shops, but I have found an Australian wholesaler and importer by searching online. Their core clientele are massage professionals and aromatherapists, so they offer oils in multiple sizes.

I started using CLARY SAGE in a diffuser on my desk when I was researching and developing the HUNGER HERO DIET. The familiar woody scent triggered memories of relaxing aromatherapy massages. It made me want to breathe deeply, and it had a calming effect.

According to the books on essential oils, clary sage may help relieve back pain, cramps, sore muscles, and headaches. Added to a warm compress, it may help soothe eye strain too. I can't tell you if it was just the scent memory that triggered the calming effect, or properties of the oil itself, but I felt less stressed and more emotionally balanced.

Feeling more relaxed, I was less likely to become agitated and fall into the trap of overeating to satisfy emotional needs. I knew that emotional eating was my biggest challenge, so I used clary sage every day. To increase the effect, I dabbed a tiny drop onto the warm pulse points at my wrists and temples. By adding this little trick into my toolbox of self-help, I think it helped me stay on track. I don't know if it will have the same effect on you, but it's worth a try.

The undiluted oil can be too strong for tender skin, so be on the safe side and add a tiny drop into a carrier oil such as body lotion. Use this perfumed cream at pulse points (temples, throat, wrists) so that the aroma can surround you. Or you can add a drop of the oil to water in a diffuser to make your environment feel a little less stressful.

There are lots of oils and blends available but only buy top quality 'pure essential oils' and not the second-grade oils offered through party plans. If you can, try before you buy. Close your eyes as you smell each one, and if it makes you want to breathe deeply, then that's the one for you. It may or may not possess intrinsic medicinal qualities, but it doesn't hurt to give it a go. Clary sage works for me, but you might prefer bergamot, jasmine, lavender, or something else. Find one that works for you, as a calm mind will help you stay on track. Be open to trying new things.

Vagus nerve stimulation

The vagus nerve relays sensory information throughout the body from the brain. This meandering nerve is the longest and most complex of the 12 cranial nerves. It helps regulate heart rate, blood pressure, digestion, speech, and sweating, and plays a balancing role in inflammation and stress management.

Recent studies implicate the vagus nerve in 'sickness behaviour' when the body is in an inflammatory state, with symptoms of fatigue, pain, poor concentration, lethargy, depression, anxiety, appetite changes, and reduced motivation (Simmons et al., 2016).

Electrical stimulation of the vagus nerve is used with some success to treat people with major depression who are not seeing improvements with medications or other types of therapy (Howland, 2014).

Something you can do at home is apply gentle but firm pressure with your fingertips **'pressure points' at the base of**

the skull, pressing for a few seconds. Follow with a gentle massage to the sides of the neck and behind the ears.

Move it or lose it

At my heaviest, I was in so much pain that I had trouble with the most basic activities of life. I struggled with showering and dressing, I couldn't reach my feet to pull on a pair of socks, or tie my shoelaces. Household chores became a major exercise in creativity, to find ways of doing things without bending down or staying on my feet for too long. If your BMI is over 40, you will know what I'm talking about.

There is a saying: "If you don't use it, you will lose it." And that is so true. If you don't use your body enough, your 'range of motion' will be limited to what you do most of the time – sitting in a chair or lying down. Joints, muscles, and ligaments become stiff and inflexible, which leads to chronic pain and makes things worse.

But when you start to lose weight, you will want to start moving. You will feel more energised, and you will want to get out and start doing things again. But be warned. If you haven't been maintaining your body properly, everything will hurt, and you risk injuring yourself.

So, before it's too late, start preparing your body for all the things you want to do once you start losing weight.

Protect your skeleton; gently stretch and flex to give your joints, muscles and ligaments a wakeup call. Aim to improve your strength and flexibility.

Flex those muscles, wiggle those fingers and toes, gently stretch – reaching up, down, and to each side – turn your head to the left then the right. If you want to, you can start doing all these movements while sitting in a chair, so don't give me excuses. Even if you can't be bothered, do it anyway. Regular physical activity such as stretching, walking, gardening, or housework can help too, just to keep the body moving.

If you have access to a swimming pool, get into it a few times a week if you can. Anything you do in the water is non-weightbearing, so the weight of your body is taken off your joints. That makes it an excellent environment for getting your body moving, but don't overdo it. All you need is 20 or 30 minutes of gentle stretching and other movements to get those joints lubricated from the inside. If you don't have a proper swimsuit, it's quite ok these days to wear a t-shirt and a pair of shorts. Get creative. Find a way. You will sleep better too.

Chapter 12: Secrets of success

Congratulations. You have come a long way, and are now at the pointy end of this process. Have you enjoyed the ride so far? We have covered so many topics:

- obesity-related health issues,
- bariatric surgical procedures and risks,
- traditional foods in countries with low rates of obesity,
- trendy diets, medical diets, and official dietary guidelines,
- macronutrients, micronutrients, and functional foods,
- latest research into gut microbiota and gut-brain axis,
- link between obesity, inflammation, and depression,
- psychology of food and why we eat too much,
- our conditioned responses,
- Antecedents, Behaviours, and Consequences,
- alternate responses that make us feel good about ourselves,
- stages of change and setting effective goals.

Everything thus far has led, like a trail of breadcrumbs, to a better understanding of your personal challenges, and HOW and WHY this HUNGER HERO DIET works so well.

- We offered insights into the physiology and psychology of WHY we eat too much,
- We provided practical tools to help you prepare for Change,
- We gave examples of exercises you can do to better understand your own personal triggers, and
- We encouraged you to look at circumventing old habits by thinking of alternate ways of responding to stress.

You now know more than most people about the latest science of obesity and weight loss, so it is time to put it all into practice.

Follow the Rules

The HUNGER HERO DIET plan is both effective and sustainable if you practice a little patience, follow the rules, and maintain a balanced diet. The weeks will fly by and the kilos will disappear. But if you are tempted to ignore the rules and substitute your own favourite foods for the ones in the plan, be warned; you will not lose weight. All the foods in this diet are there for a reason; they are not random choices.

Once you lose the first 10 kilos you can start introducing more variety in your food choices and cooking methods… but until then, just follow the rules.

If you hate rules, it might help to think of them as INSIDER SECRETS. Call them what you will, but ignore them at your peril. Prepare to challenge yourself. Every rule is there for a reason. If you pick and choose, you will fail. To lose weight you need to follow ALL the rules, not just those you like.

This revolutionary diet plan is nutritionally balanced, portion-controlled, and includes foods to curb your appetite. These special foods are your HUNGER HEROES. Not only are they good for you, but they will satisfy cravings for sweet, savoury, sour, salty, crunchy, smooth, creamy, and spicy. In ways that will amaze you, the core ingredients work together to suppress your appetite and lift your mood.

If you are serious about wanting to change how you feel about yourself, you need to accept the truth: What you have been doing is not working for you, and you need help. Accept that you don't have all the answers, and commit to learning new skills. Be prepared to relinquish some old beliefs and trust in the science. And above all, do not cut corners. Follow ALL the rules.

Life can improve, and it's never too late. Become the best version of yourself. You can do this!

RULE 1: Tick tock, watch the clock

Most diets encourage you to eat frequent small meals throughout the day to reduce sugar spikes and avoid hunger, but that advice is FALSE. People who follow this 'grazing' style of eating tend to consume more food and more calories, especially calorie-dense snacks later in the day, and into the evening. Women, in particular, are more likely to be overweight or obese if they follow a grazing pattern (Leech et al., 2017).

We need to reduce the frequency of feeds, and change our approach to eating. By only eating at specific times, you won't be thinking about food all the time, and you will give your gut a much-needed holiday. Remember, a happy gut can help achieve a healthier mind and body.

Time-restricted feeding and fasting (TRFF) requires a period of voluntary abstinence from all types of food or drink that contain calories. There are many ways you can do this, but studies have found the 16:8 form of intermittent fasting is:

- the most effective for significant weight loss and better metabolic health,
- far superior to the 5:2 or 'alternate day' methods, and
- having a positive impact on gut microbiota (Patterson and Sears, 2017).

In the HUNGER HERO DIET, you will follow the 16:8 protocol. You will fast for 16 hours every day, and consume all your calories in the remaining 8 hours.

Realistically, it shouldn't be that difficult to avoid food for 16 hours, as most of us are asleep for 7-9 hours anyway. It can take a while to break the habit of looking for food as soon as you wake up, but we have a few tricks for you. Just stick to the diet and you'll soon wonder why you ever needed to eat so early in the morning. If you follow the same routine every day, you quickly develop this new behaviour into a comfortable habit, so it soon becomes your new normal.

By delaying your first meal until later in the day you can reduce your daily calorie intake by up to 500 calories, which can potentially add up to 3,500 calories over a week – which equates to losing half a kilo of fat, just by skipping breakfast and morning tea. But to make it work, you must not consume any calories for the entire 16-hr fast. Interestingly, a prolonged morning fast does not increase your appetite later in the day, so you will not feel compelled to overeat at lunch time to make up for a missed breakfast.

16:8 is the most effective form of intermittent fasting for weight loss

Prolonging the nightly fasting state has many clinical benefits. Data from the National Health and Nutrition Examination Surveys (NHANES) shows that:
- each 3-hour increase in night-time fasting duration is associated with a reduced risk of type 2 diabetes, and
- women who consumed most of their food later in the day, but before 5pm, had lower levels of C-reactive protein (CRP), a blood marker for systemic inflammation (Patterson and Sears, 2017).

A 7-year follow-up of 2,337 breast cancer survivors in the Women's Healthy Eating and Living Study (WHEL) found that those who fasted LESS than 13 hours per night had a higher risk of recurrent cancer (Patterson and Sears, 2017), which suggests a 16-hr fast has significant health benefits.

To follow the HUNGER HERO DIET,
1. Choose an 8-hr window of opportunity, when you eat all your meals and snack for the day,
2. Decide on specific times within that 8-hr window for 2 meals and 2 snacks,
3. Watch the clock and only eat at those specific times. (This helps to reprogram your body clock to only expect food at those times. It will help you avoid opportunistic

eating just because something is available, and it will stop you thinking about food all the time.),
4. For the remaining 16-hr fast, abstain from consuming anything containing calories. But you will be encouraged to rehydrate each morning with water, tea, and other fluids. These drinks will be explained in the next chapter.
5. Every day, after fasting for 16 hours (including sleep), you will have a remaining 8-hour window for 2 main meals and 2 snacks.

For example,
- my first meal of the day (break-fast) is at 11.30am,
- followed by an afternoon snack at 2.30pm,
- evening meal at 5.30-6pm, and
- evening snack/dessert at 7pm.

These times were right for me because I have always been hungry later in the day, especially in the evening while watching TV, and research tells us that most overweight people have the same problem.

You might need a different 8-hour block to suit your lifestyle and other commitments. For example, if you're working in an office, you might find 12 noon, 3pm, 6pm, and 8pm suit you better. These feeding times are not rigid, but you need to develop a consistent routine.

The 24-hour light–dark cycle influences food intake, energy usage, and weight control. Shift workers who eat at night have an increased risk of obesity, as the abnormal hours affect the appetite-regulating hormones. If you can, try to eat most meals during the day.

RULE 2: Repeat, repeat, repeat

REPETITION is key to building any new skill or behaviour.

When we get behind the wheel of a car, we don't consciously think about how to drive the car. We have done it so many times before, repeated the set of manoeuvres over and over, to a point where driving becomes almost instinctive. If we need to stop, we instinctively brake; we don't have to think about lifting our foot and pressing down on the pedal. We need to stay aware of what we're doing, but we don't have to think about every little thing before we do it.

Shopping for food and preparing meals should be just as easy. By repeating the same behaviours over and over, they soon become second nature.

You won't be thinking about food all the time, wondering what to have for dinner, what's in the fridge, or what you need to buy. Your shopping list will be simple and food preparation will become easy, natural, and quick. With the minimum effort, you will have everything you need – in your pantry, freezer, and fridge. You won't be thinking, "I can't be bothered", then grab a pizza on the way home, only to kick yourself later on.

Routine is crucial; it takes food-related thoughts out of your mind and stops your mouth from salivating. If you don't think about food, you won't be tempted to go onto autopilot and head to the fridge. Even as you read this, your mind is now on food and you're probably thinking about what is in your fridge. See how easily triggered we are?

The best advice I can give you is to stick to the same daily menu for the first few weeks, so you're not looking in the fridge and wondering "What's for dinner?". Every month or so, you can try adding a new dish to your repertoire, if you like. But you must stick to the core ingredients of the diet.

Repetition is necessary to create new healthy habits. Repeat the SAME behaviours at the SAME time every day, and under the SAME conditions. You can rewire your brain with a healthy routine., but new habits can take 6 months to become automatic, so give it time.

You can lose a few kilos if you follow a fad diet for the usual 4, 6, 8 or 12-weeks, but you need closer to 6 months to create new habits, ow the weight will always come back.

This is why you need to follow the HUNGER HERO DIET for at least 6 months, to reinforce all the new behaviours – to lose weight every week, consistently, and keep it off. If you persist, you will avoid falling back into old habits that see you regaining all the weight you lost. Create a routine, then repeat, repeat, repeat. It is that simple.

RULE 3: Be mindful – stay focused

You have the power over how YOU react and respond to THIS MOMENT in your life. Focus on NOW – TODAY, not yesterday, not tomorrow. Become mindful of what you are feeling RIGHT HERE, RIGHT NOW. If you can do this EVERY DAY, tomorrow will look after itself.

That is the powerful simplicity of what behavioural scientists call 'Mindfulness' – being FULLY AWARE in the moment, not distracted by what is happening around you, by other people, by the past, or the future. And don't be distracted by your own erratic thoughts. Don't let the noisy chatter of what Buddhists call your 'monkey mind' undermine your concentration and resolve. Control those thoughts and stay focussed on the task in front of you. Give it your FULL ATTENTION. Be fully present in the NOW.

With practice, your breathing will become more regulated, and you will feel a sense of calm wash over you. This can have an amazing effect on your digestion and help protect you from eating too much. Such a simple practice, but with enormous results.

Avoid sensory cues

Mindfulness is your friend; 'mindless eating' is your enemy.

Every time you walk past the fridge or pantry you are at risk of mindless eating – eating without being consciously aware of what you are about to do, or the consequences; running on autopilot, following unconscious cues to behave in a conditioned manner.

Seeing an ad on TV for food, or just sitting down to watch a movie – can be cues to start thinking about snacks. And if you don't drag your mind away, the thoughts of food get stronger and stronger. You feel driven to get up and raid the kitchen pantry. So easily, you could scoff an entire packet of crisps, a block of chocolate, or a tub of ice-cream.

You must avoid those sensory cues at all costs. If we see it or smell it, we will want to eat it. Just like the family dog, we begin to salivate.

You must **AVOID TEMPTATION** :
- LOOK AWAY from the TV when the ads come on, and stop watching cooking shows.
- Avoid supermarket aisles where all the sweet and savoury treats are on display.

- Avoid watching others eating and drinking (especially when out shopping), and
- Always shop with a list, to avoid impulse buying.

Be mindful... as you prepare food

When the time comes to prepare your food, give it your undivided attention. Don't be distracted by people, technology, or noise. Try to be fully present in the moment. Immerse yourself in the pleasure of the moment, and stick to the plan:

1. Prepare all meals and snacks in the kitchen, but DO NOT eat there.
2. Be mindful as you choose food from the fridge and pantry.
3. Place all ingredients on the kitchen bench BEFORE you begin constructing your meal (or snack). This will allow you to visualise the meal you are about to prepare, and help you to stick to the correct portion sizes.
4. Be mindful as you prepare the food. If you can, sit quietly on a kitchen stool up at the bench. Relax. Don't rush it. Take your time.
5. Don't nibble as you go. Practice restraint. (Remember, you're not allowed to eat anything in the kitchen.)
6. Try to arrange your food on a plate so it looks attractive and appetising. It will taste better if it looks good. And for the first few weeks, take a quick photo of every meal. (Knowing that you're going to record your food makes you more accountable, and less likely to overdo the portions. I also found that by arranging the food properly on the plate, and taking a photo, I was fully aware of every bit of food on the plate. It made me eat more slowly, savouring every mouthful, and had a

positive effect on appetite control. It might sound daft, but give it a go.)
7. To practice another bit of delayed gratification, clean up the kitchen and put everything else away in the pantry and fridge before you start eating. Don't leave anything sitting out until later, as this can be a sensory cue to get you thinking of food again!
8. Now leave the kitchen. Take your meal/snack into another room, preferably to a spot on a table which is specifically set aside as the place to eat. For most people, this would be a dining table.
9. Sit down at the table. Look at the food on your plate. Admire how it looks. Think about how it will taste, the textures and the smell. Engage all your senses in the moment. Don't be distracted by anything else. Enjoy every mouthful.

Be mindful... as you eat

WHERE you eat is as important as HOW you eat. Mindless snacking occurs if you eat in the kitchen, your bedroom, the living room, out on the balcony, in the garden, or at the computer.

- NEVER eat in the kitchen or at the kitchen bench.
- Do not eat in the lounge room, in front of the TV, at the computer, while reading, or while distracted by others.
- If you're at work, do not eat at your desk. Find somewhere else to sit and eat, away from distractions.

There is only ONE PLACE you can eat, and that must be away from the kitchen. Allocate completely separate spaces in your home for food preparation and eating. This intentional behaviour helps to prevent 'mindless' snacking or overeating (which can happen if you eat in the kitchen, your bedroom, the living room, out on the balcony, in the garden, or at the computer).

Most of us have a dining room table, or another table and chairs away from the kitchen, so get into the habit of ONLY EATING when seated at that table. Have it permanently set up as a place to eat, and avoid using it for anything else. Choose a chair where you cannot see the television. If possible, make it a spot with natural light and a view to nature – aspects that help keep you calm and improve your mood. If you can stay calm and relaxed, you are less likely to overeat.

Take your time, eat slowly, focus on the food... and indulge your senses

When you start eating, focus on your plate, enjoying the look, smell and taste of every mouthful. Is it sweet, sour, crunchy, creamy, smooth, firm, aromatic? Concentrate on the sensations of every mouthful. Take your time. Eat slowly and mindfully. Enjoy the moment. Congratulate yourself for being so disciplined.

When practical to do so, eat with your hands or use chopsticks. By eating in this very tactile way, you will be more aware of what you are about to eat, and will put less in your mouth. Keep looking at the food as you eat; don't look away. You will eat more slowly and eat less. Chopsticks might sound like a gimmick, but Asian countries have the lowest obesity rates, so they must be doing something right.

RULE 4: Size does matter

PORTION CONTROL is something you must learn to do properly, and continue practicing for the rest of your life – if you want to lose weight and keep it off.

We get fat because we eat too much, even if we make healthy choices. But nobody wants to be measuring their food at every meal, so you need a couple of simple tricks:

- Store high-calorie foods in single serves (in the pantry, freezer, fridge), and
- Use smaller plates and bowls for all your meals and snacks.

Store food in single serves

As you will soon discover, the recommended foods in this diet are economical and available in the larger supermarkets. This was intentional, making the foods accessible and affordable for most people.

Where possible, the foods are packaged in single serves, or a single serve is easily determined without having to weigh or measure anything. This is especially true for the snacks.

- For foods you buy by the kilo, such as fresh seafood or steak, divide them into individual portion sizes as soon as you get home. Using digital kitchen scales, aim for a portion size of just under 200g for your seafood and meat (and that includes the weight of the shells on prawns). Sandwich-size resealable plastic bags are ideal for storing these portions in the fridge or freezer.
- When storing portions in the freezer, remove as much air as you can from the plastic bags before sealing them,

then lay them as flat as possible when stacking in the freezer.
- Always store raw and cooked food on separate shelves in the fridge and in separate sections of the freezer. This avoids cross-contamination, but it also simplifies food preparation. When the pack thaws, you know exactly what to expect.

By taking a few minutes when you get home from shopping, you will not have to measure anything when you go to prepare a meal. Once you know what a single serve looks like, you can sit back and relax. No more guess work. No more mistakes. Train your brain to recognise portion sizes.

Plates, bowls and cutlery

Dinner plates from the early 1900s were half the size they are today, so we need to learn from that. Most Asian cultures use small plates and bowls, and chopsticks, and in Japan, the custom has always been to eat slowly. The aim is to enjoy your food, be aware of how much you are eating, and establish a healthy rhythm of regular mealtimes.

- For main meals, use smaller plates. Arrange your food so that every piece lies flat on that plate. By not stacking your food, you are maintaining portion control, and it will look like a large serve – helping to satisfy your appetite sooner.
- For fruit and desserts, use a coffee cup or a tiny bowl that can only fit one cup of food. This encourages portion control, and helps you visualise what a single portion looks like.
- Don't try to squeeze extra food onto your plate; it's not clever or funny; and the only person you're fooling is

yourself. If your meal doesn't fit easily across the plate, or your dessert doesn't fit comfortably into a cup, your portions are too big.

- For the first few weeks, photograph every plate of food you prepare; pretend they are going to be seen in a magazine. This will discourage you from cheating with portion sizes or ingredients, and if the food looks good, it will be more satisfying.

RULE 5: Keep track with your DIET DIARY

Keep a daily food diary and record your weight

Every day, in your DIET DIARY,
- Write the day and date
- Record your WEIGHT
- Record everything you EAT and DRINK, and the TIME
- If something comes to mind, comment on your how you are feeling, as this will help ground you in the moment.

Your reasons for wanting to lose weight are not only physical, but emotional too. You might be feeling vulnerable at this point, but now is the time to face facts and move forward. To help you do that, we are showing you ways to keep track of your progress – daily, weekly, and monthly. Studies have proven that people who keep food diaries lose much more weight, so it makes sense to be one of those people.

Record keeping is crucial to your weight loss success. Seeing all the food written down in front of you helps your conscious mind realise you should not be feeling hungry, and hopefully convey that message to your gut. And by noting the TIME, you will know when to have your next meal or snack, and when to begin your fast.

Chart your weight loss (weekly and monthly)

Seeing tangible evidence of progress is a strong motivator to stay on track and keep going. How will you track your progress and measure your success? How will you know if you are losing weight?

- Record your BASELINE measurements before you start:

   Weight (in kilograms), and Height (in metres).
- Weigh yourself without clothes first thing EVERY MORNING and record it in your DIET DIARY, against the day's date. (On this same page, you will be recording everything you eat throughout the day, and the time of day that you eat.)
- A free phone app like **WeightFit®** will do all these calculations for you. Simply enter your weight into the app every morning. It's free to download onto your phone.

The simplest way to chart your progress is to use a phone app. But you can use an Excel spreadsheet (with a graph), or even a piece of paper if you prefer. Here's the way to create a simple chart, starting with your BASELINE measurements, and checking progress every 4 weeks.

Measure	Baseline	4 weeks	8 weeks	12 weeks	16 weeks
Height (m)	1.7m(170cm)				
Weight (kg)	120 kg	112kg	108kg	104kg	100kg
BMI	42	38.8	37.4	36	34.6

Weight can fluctuate day to day, so only use the DAILY weight as a guide. To gain a more meaningful view of your progress, look at weekly and monthly changes in your weight and BMI. (And, if you like, take a photo every few weeks and compare.)

Chart improvements to Quality of Life (QoL)

Physical measurements are not the only measure of success. The emotional and psychological benefits of successful weight loss are as important as the physical ones, and many of these will be your secondary goals.

Let these questions prompt you, then open your **DIET DIARY** and jot down a few answers:
- What negative feelings do you have about being overweight?
- How does obesity impact on your life?
- Is your health suffering?
- Is your social life almost non-existent?
- Are you struggling with normal daily activities?
- Are financial matters causing you to worry?
- Are your relationships under stress?

Using your answers, jot down a few examples of SIMPLE TASKS you struggle to do, or things that you feel are stopping you from enjoying life. (See the example below, then follow the instructions to create your own chart.)

Create your own QoL progress chart:
- Open your **DIET DIARY** and create a chart with columns, as you can see in the example.

- List the issues you currently have around being overweight. You might 5 or 25. Some will be more important to you than others, but list them all.
- Assign a value to each one, using a simple scale of 1 (it's not a problem) to 10 (it's a huge problem). This is your baseline data (starting point).
- Reassess every few weeks, and record the new value. Some values will show improvement faster than others, but as you lose weight, recognising even the smallest change in QoL will make you feel so much better about yourself.

How I feel	Base line score	After 4 weeks	After 8 weeks	After 12 weeks	After 16 weeks
Struggle to breathe	10	8	7	6	4
Exhausted every day	10	8	6	5	4
Too fat for outings	10	9	8	6	3
Can't wear nice clothes	10	10	9	8	7
Struggle to reach toes	10	10	9	8	5
It hurts to walk	10	10	8	6	5

When you see improvements in these scores, you will know for sure that your quality of life is improving. And for most of us, this is the real reason we want to lose weight. We desperately want to feel better about ourselves and more able to live a normal life.

I had favourite clothes that were too small. When I could finally wear them comfortably, I had achieved one of my secondary goals. They became my most meaningful weight loss guide.

RULE 6: Follow the Rules

REMOVE TEMPTATION :
- Clear out the pantry, fridge, and freezer of foods you want to avoid. Give them away, or pack them away – just get rid of them. Out of sight, out of mind.
- Replace them with all the foods you have decided to include in your new diet.
- Rearrange your food storage to help you choose the right foods at the right time, such as keeping your healthy snacks within easy reach in the fridge or pantry.

FOLLOW THE RULES :
- Maintain a **DIET DIARY**.
- Record everything you eat and drink, and the time – until your new behaviours and routines become automatic.
- Record your progress with daily weight and weekly milestones.
- Practice portion control. Where you can, store your protein foods and snacks in individual portions, so you don't have to think about it every day. Make it easy on yourself.
- Avoid sensory stimuli and temptation.
- Do NOT think about food when you are NOT EATING.
- Only think about food while eating or preparing food.
- Go shopping early in the day when your resolve is strong, and always use a **SHOPPING LIST**.

- Add items to your shopping list only after you have eaten.
- Favourite clothes that don't fit? Try them on every few weeks. They will be your best measure of success.
- Keep track and get snapping; take lots of photos of yourself and your food.
- Practice self-care.

Old habits die hard, so if you find yourself standing in front of the fridge with the door open, pour yourself a big glass of cold water and sip on it until the urge has passed. Get out of the kitchen.

Never eat in the kitchen

- Water is your best friend. Keep sipping on it throughout the day, especially during the morning fast.
- Throughout the day, distract your 'monkey mind' with activities that are not food related. Read a book, watch a movie, call a friend, start writing a journal, go for a swim, go for a walk, or go back to sleep! Whatever it takes, keep your mind away from food.
- Only think about food when you ARE supposed to be eating or preparing food.
- Avoid temptation; look away, walk away.

Ok, it might seem like a lot of rules, but here are the basics to guide you on the road to success, and beyond:
- Maintain portion control.
- Maintain regular mealtimes.
- Do not restrict food groups.

- Plan ahead, stock your fridge, freezer, and pantry with the right foods.
- Keep your body moving, with as much normal daily activity as you can comfortably achieve, and practice gentle stretches to maintain flexibility and function.

Mindfulness is your friend; 'mindless eating' is your enemy.

Chapter 13: Hunger Hero
MENU PLAN

PORTION CONTROL is key, and I give you simple ways to manage it. Most of the supermarket foods are pre-packaged or individually wrapped. This is especially important when choosing high energy snack foods. Once you know what a single serve looks like, you can sit back and relax. You won't be spending your day counting calories!

STICK TO A SET **ROUTINE** for meals and snacks, and arm yourself with a pre-arranged set of calorie-controlled foods to choose from. You will lose weight, and still experience all the pleasures of eating.

ROUTINE AND **REPETITION** are necessary when trying to develop new habits. This is why LUNCH and DINNER are very similar. Don't worry; this won't always be the case. But you need to start out this way to get your mind off food. You won't be spending your days planning meals, shopping for additional foods, or binging. Importantly, by repeating the same food preparation at every meal, you will quickly develop new behaviours that soon become effortless and automatic.

SMART SNACKS will help you stay on track. When you want creamy, you'll get creamy. When you want spicy, you'll get spicy. When you want a yummy salty crunch, you will know how to get it. These are the flavours and textures that give us pleasure, which make food so much fun. You don't have to give up any of these taste sensations, but you do need to learn how to make better choices. And once you discover these foods, you can forget all about calorie counting.

If you **PLAN AHEAD**, you will have lots of simple options to satisfy any desire you might have for favourite flavours and textures. Just keep your fridge, freezer and pantry stocked with the right things. It is so easy, and I am about to share it with you. The **LET'S GO SHOPPING** chapter provides a shopping list for your convenience.

Nutritionally balanced, portion controlled... with foods to satisfy cravings, and lift your mood

The HUNGER HERO MENU PLAN is deceptively simple, but effective. Once you master the basics, you will begin to experiment with different combinations and flavours. This is where the magic happens. This is why this diet plan is so sustainable for the long-term. Once you understand the principles, you can keep adding to your personal repertoire of fast, easy, and incredibly healthy food that tastes amazing and makes you feel fantastic. So, let's get started.

Morning fast and cleanse

Remember RULE #1... Tick, tock, watch the clock. This morning fast and cleanse begins from when you wake up, until lunchtime. This creates a total overnight fasting period of 16 hours, including sleep. Importantly, mornings are for rehydrating; replacing fluids and flushing toxins, without adding calories. Throughout the morning, you will be drinking:

- 2 -3 glasses of chilled water, with a teaspoon of apple cider vinegar in each glass, and
- 1-2 cups of spiced black tea (organic Chai, no milk or sugar)

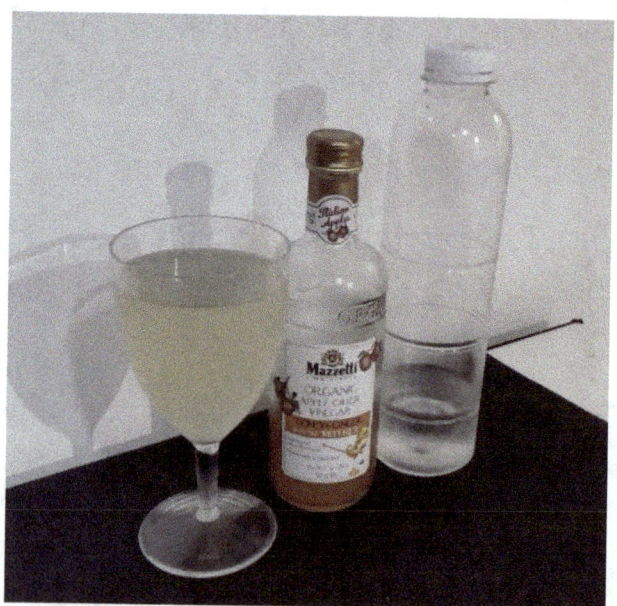

Figure 2: Apple cider vinegar in cold water

- Start the day by slowly drinking a glass of COLD WATER to which you have added a teaspoon of APPLE CIDER VINEGAR. Sip it slowly and savour the unique flavour. The slight sourness of the water will target the saliva inside your mouth and curb any immediate desire for food. If you can, repeat again later in the morning, as it will help you stretch the fast until lunch.
- Across the morning, enjoy one or two cups of hot 'CHAI TEA' (spiced black tea) without milk or sugar. Avoid calories before lunch. My favourite is Nature's Cuppa organic chai spiced tea – black tea bags, spiced with a combination of cinnamon, cardamon, ginger, cloves, black pepper, and pure vanilla bean. It has a warm spicy flavour and 'appetite suppressing' effect on the mouth.

Sorry, NO COFFEE. It has too many associations. When we have a morning coffee, what else do we normally do? Reach for a cigarette, a pastry, toast, or a bacon and egg roll? And at that mid-morning break do we look for the biscuits to go with the coffee? Get the idea? When we have a coffee, we have a conditioned response to expect food, so we need to avoid it (for now).

Lunch: 11.30am-12 noon

- 3x RICE PAPER ROLLS with TINNED TUNA, Greek yoghurt, chili, pickled sushi ginger, fresh herbs and coleslaw salad vegetables (see **RECIPE** section).
- To kickstart your weight loss each week, try to start the week with 2 days where you substitute PRAWNS for the tuna. You need to buy prawns in the shell and peel them yourself. This is very important.

This is when you break-the-fast, with your first meal of the day; more of a brunch than a normal lunch. Don't wait until you start feeling hungry. You can start preparing the food anytime after 11am. But pace yourself. **Once you start eating, your 8-hr feeding time begins.** For example, if you start eating at 11.30am, your afternoon snack should be around 2.30pm, your dinner near 5.30pm, and your evening snack at 7pm. By creating this routine, you will develop new healthy habits and suppress your appetite.

These Vietnamese-inspired gluten-free rice paper rolls are a perfect combination of flavours and textures – smooth, chewy, creamy, sour, spicy, crunchy, sweet and aromatic. They contain all the food groups, with the added benefit of being prebiotic (coleslaw) and probiotic (natural Greek yoghurt).

The core ingredient is seafood, which is low calorie and high in nutrients. Most days it will be TINNED TUNA (packed in springwater, not brine or oil), and on other days you will use PRAWNS.

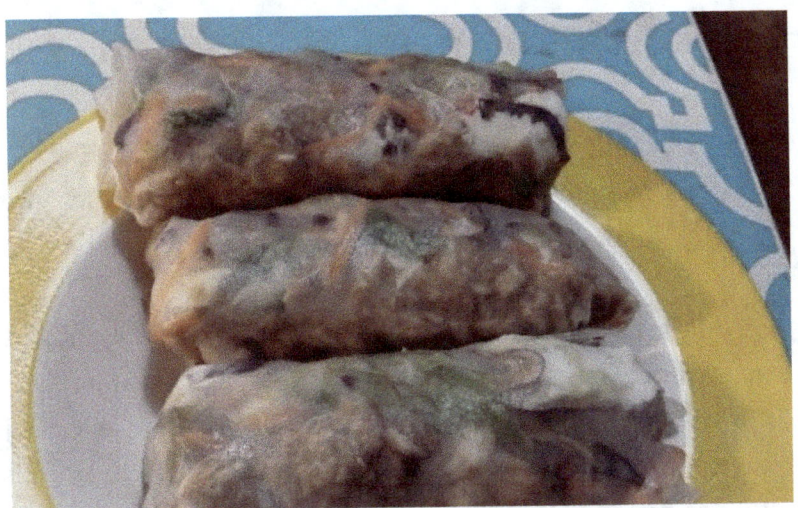
Figure 3: Rice paper rolls with tuna salad

There is something quite special about these rice paper rolls when they have large juicy prawns inside them; after eating them, you feel completely full! This recipe creates a balanced meal, low in calories, and high in nutrients, but I am yet to discover the secret to why these prawn rolls are such HUNGER HEROES.

From personal experience, this food combination only works as an appetite suppressor when encased in rice papers – which is a surprising and exciting discovery.

Check the **RECIPE** chapter for lots of variations.

Afternoon snack : 2.30pm

- 3x THIN RICE CAKES with COTTAGE CHEESE, and
- A mouthful of sauerkraut to curb hunger, if required. Do not underestimate how effective this can be.

HINT: For a sour hit between meals, try a mouthful of sauerkraut. Get the jar out of the fridge, and with a fork, dig into the packed mound of pickled cabbage and extract just enough for a mouthful. Eat it slowly and savour it. Do this as often as needed. **The sourness will alter the enzymes in your mouth, so you won't be feeling hungry**. It keeps your mouth happy! This works in the same way as the apple cider vinegar in the morning. It's a great trick. It's so simple, but it works a treat!

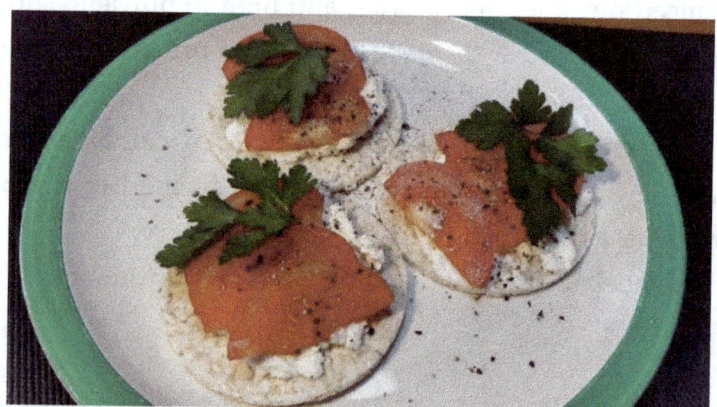

Figure 4: Rice cakes with cottage cheese and tomato

To keep your mouth happy, add a few extra flavours to the cottage cheese now and then, such as sliced tomato or cucumber. Check the **RECIPE** chapter for inspiration.

SMART SNACKS are the answer to mid-afternoon or evening munchies. They are pre-portioned foods or drinks chosen for their LOW CALORIE content, their ability to SATISFY whatever textural sensation or flavour bomb your MOUTH is wanting, and their inherent nutrient value. Eat ONE smart snack mid-afternoon and ONE after dinner.

Smart snacks can be sweet, savoury, crunchy, or creamy. Fruit is the obvious sweet choice, and yoghurt is creamy. Rice cakes and crackers provide a good crunch.

If your mouth wants something sweet, give it fruit instead of chocolate. If it wants something crunchy, give it rice cakes or rice crackers, instead of potato chips. If it wants something creamy, give it Greek yoghurt instead of ice-cream or custard!

Dinner: 5.30-6pm

- 3x RICE PAPER ROLLS with PAN-SEARED TUNA STEAK or PAN-SEARED WHITE FISH, with Greek yoghurt, chili, pickled sushi ginger, fresh herbs and coleslaw salad vegetables (see **RECIPE** SECTION)

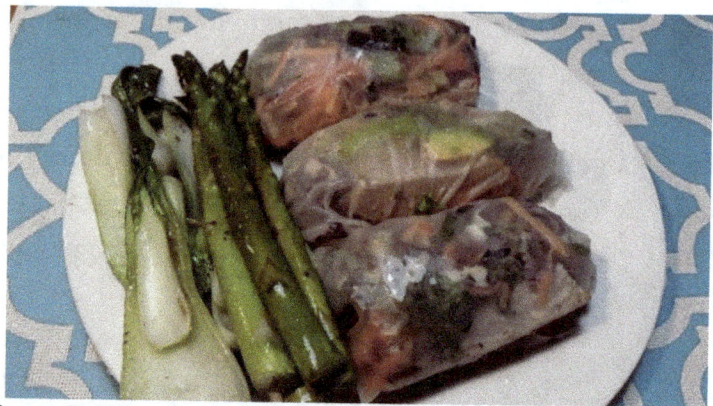

Figure 5: Rice paper rolls with seared tuna steak or white fish

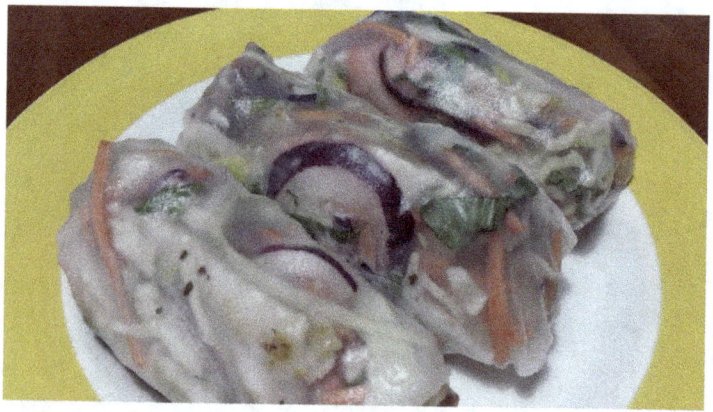

These fish fillets will live in your freezer. You buy them in packs of individually-wrapped portions from the

supermarket. The **LET'S GO SHOPPING** chapter provides the details.

Check out the **RECIPE** chapter for winter and summer variations – salads, soups, noodles, and lots of yummy vegetables.

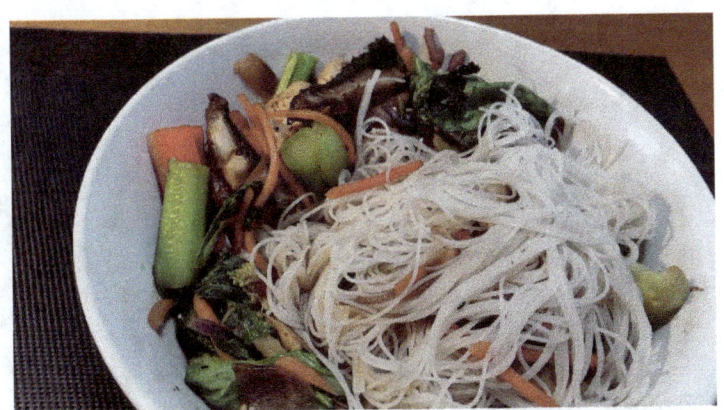

Figure 6: Sauteed veg with mushrooms and noodles

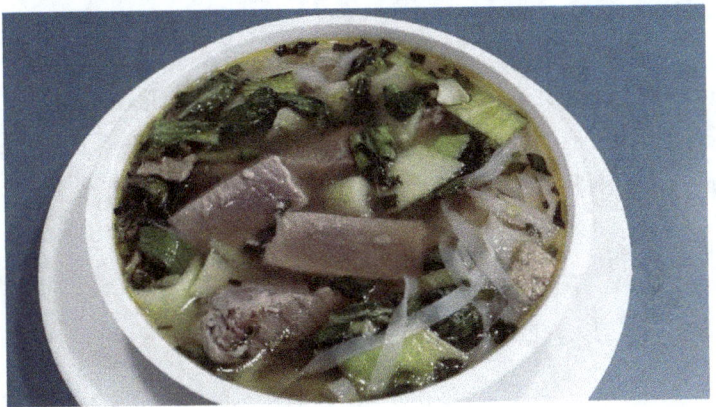

Evening snack : 7-7.30pm

- 2 tablespoons of bottled Morello cherries with 2 tablespoons of full-fat Greek yoghurt, and
- Caffeine-free herbal tea, if desired (e.g., chamomile, peppermint)

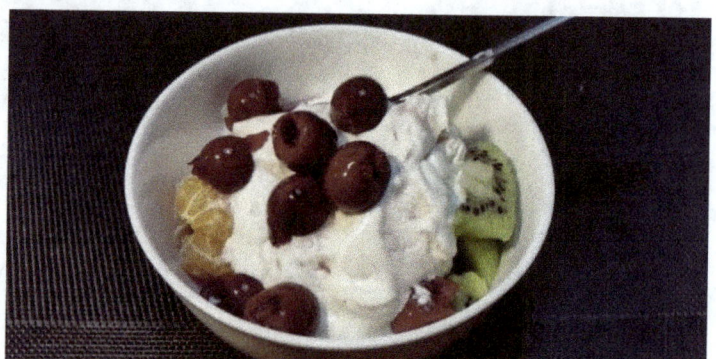

Figure 7: Yoghurt with Morello cherries (fresh seasonal fruit is optional)

Again, SMART SNACKS are the key to low-calorie appetite control with nutritional value. Check out the **RECIPE** section for lots of sweet and savoury variations to suit whatever your mouth is wanting.

Chapter 14: The HUNGER HEROES

Most of the foods in the HUNGER HERO DIET are **FUNCTIONAL FOODS**, which means they provide special health benefits above and beyond basic nutrition. The core elements are deceptively simple – seafood, Greek yoghurt, rice products, fruit, and vegetables – with a few extras thrown in now and then, just to keep it interesting.

Many of these foods are HUNGER HEROES, and they elevate this diet to something extraordinary. Not only are they good for us, but they have a remarkable ability to subdue our appetite. They appear front and centre on the menu every day, in main meals and snacks, so don't skip these foods and expect to lose weight.

When developing the HUNGER HERO DIET, I intentionally used products from my local supermarket, to ensure the foods in this diet were readily accessible and economical – not just for me, but for you too. I used the supermarket brands whenever possible, and I was delighted to find I preferred the flavour and texture of these products over the more expensive brands.

Even if you cannot leave the house, most people have access to online shopping and the major supermarkets will deliver everything you need to your kitchen bench. I had that thought front of mind when I developed this diet, and it's another huge benefit of shopping through a major supermarket chain. I want everyone to have access to the foods, and not be disadvantaged financially.

Most meals are 'constructed' from tinned or pre-packaged foods, so there is very little preparation. Even if you struggle to stand up for any length of time, you can prepare most of these meals while sitting down. How easy is that? And if you don't know how to cook, don't worry. If you can make a sandwich, you have the skills to prepare these meals.

We have not removed any food groups, but we have avoided foods that are known to trigger gut inflammation – gluten and lactose – and others that can trigger painful joint inflammation in some people, such as tomatoes and roast chicken.

I admit to not having any studies confirming the inflammatory effects of roast chicken, but from personal observation, whenever I indulge in a hot chook from the supermarket, my joints cease up and I can barely walk the next day. The same occurs when I eat tomatoes or sugary foods, so these foods are limited.

We need to listen to our bodies, even if it means removing a favourite food from our diet. I love chunky bread, fresh tomatoes, and hot roast chicken, but they don't like me, so I had to make a choice. Most people can eat fish and shellfish, but a small percentage will have an allergic reaction to shellfish. Hopefully everyone will be able to eat fish and other types of seafood, to gain the exceptional health benefits.

The foods that made it into the HUNGER HERO DIET should be well-tolerated by most people, to allow weight loss to occur in a healthy way. Pushing through all the noise and nonsense of fad diets, the strongest evidence says we should avoid doing anything drastic. We should maintain normal fat intake, cut back a little on carbs, and compensate by eating a little more protein. By making those small changes, we can 'increase 24-hour satiety, thermogenesis, sleeping energy expenditure, protein balance, and fat oxidation' (Abete et al., 2010), which means you will:

- feel less hungry,
- burn more energy,
- lose less muscle, and
- burn more fat.

Rice, not wheat

AVOID WHEAT products such as bread, pasta, and pastries. (I never lost weight while eating bread and pasta.) The gluten in wheat is known to upset the gut lining and trigger inflammation.

Products made from rice and corn are excellent gluten-free substitutes, but in the HUNGER HERO DIET we prefer to use RICE as our primary carbohydrate. RICE grain is gentle on the gut, but it is extraordinarily high in calories. Therefore, we only use products made from rice, which allow for easy PORTION CONTROL.

- RICE PAPER is made from rice flour and tapioca. We use them in much the same way as people use bread and wraps to make sandwiches. We use them to construct rice paper rolls, with fillings such as tuna, salad, and condiments.

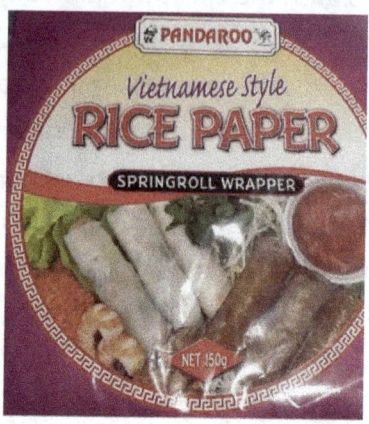

- RICE CAKES make excellent snacks. They are low in calories and provide a pleasing crunch. The THIN rice cakes have fewer calories than the thick ones, and they are easier to eat. Some are flavoured, but the plain ones lend themselves to an unlimited array of toppings. Choose whatever works best for you.
- RICE CRACKERS are a great snack too, particularly the multigrain brown rice crackers or the BBQ flavour. One row in the pack is a single serve.
- Avoid wheat-based egg noodles and look for RICE NOODLES. Packs of dried rice noodles are readily available – the thin vermicelli style or the flat ribbon variety. In the colder months, add a warming broth to your repertoire for lunch or dinner. A small single serve of rice noodles can enliven a hot Asian-style soup, or transform a bowl of tuna and salad into a tasty poke bowl.

Fermented dairy, and alternatives

Dairy products are high in essential nutrients, but many contain lactose sugars which can upset the gut and trigger inflammation. But if milk undergoes fermentation, those sugars are taken up by the live bacteria. This produces products which are almost lactose-free, and much more easily tolerated.

- Natural Greek-style yoghurt retains a tiny amount of lactose after the fermentation process, but most people can tolerate it without any problems. In fact, the residual live bacteria in natural yoghurt may have a healthy probiotic effect.
- Many cheeses undergo fermentation. Hard cheeses like parmesan, cheddar and Swiss fall into this category, but only consume very small amounts (and rarely) as they are high in calories.
- COTTAGE CHEESE is the best choice, and it makes an excellent afternoon snack when spread on thin rice cakes. Ricotta cheese can also be used.
- Instead of cow's milk, substitute a creamy alternative made from soy, rice, or almonds. I've tried all of these, and my personal preference is for SOY MILK, either in the regular, full-fat or lite versions. It has a pleasant creaminess that satisfies, and makes excellent smoothies. And recent studies have found commercially produced almond milks lack any substantial nutritional benefit, so we are better off sticking to soy milk for our calcium needs.

Seafood (fish and shellfish)

Seafood is the staple ingredient in your menu, especially tuna and prawns. Aim for at least one seafood meal every day, preferably two.

Most lunches are built around tinned tuna, whereas the evening meal can be pre-packaged frozen tuna steaks (or white fish fillets) which are thawed and pan-seared for a change of texture and flavour. You can swap the meals around, but I like having a hot evening meal. To jazz it up, I sometimes add a few greens to the pan as the tuna is cooking; they make an excellent side dish.

Regular fish consumption can help you lose weight, lower blood pressure, lower triglycerides, reduce inflammation, increase HDL cholesterol, and improve insulin/glucose regulation. The omega-3s help control appetite (by improving leptin sensitivity) (Abete et al., 2010).

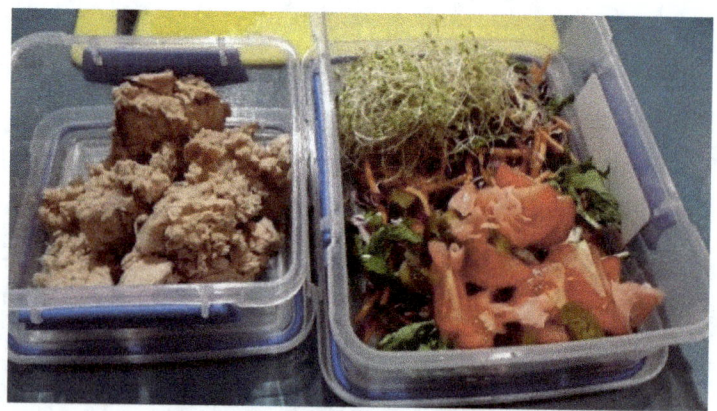

Figure 8: Tinned tuna and salad

- TUNA is an excellent source of protein, omega-3s, phosphorous, and vitamins B3, B12 and D. Yellowfin tuna is a rich source of selenium – which helps reduce inflammation and oxidative stress (free radicals). Tinned tuna is affordable and easily accessible, as are packs of individually wrapped frozen tuna steaks.

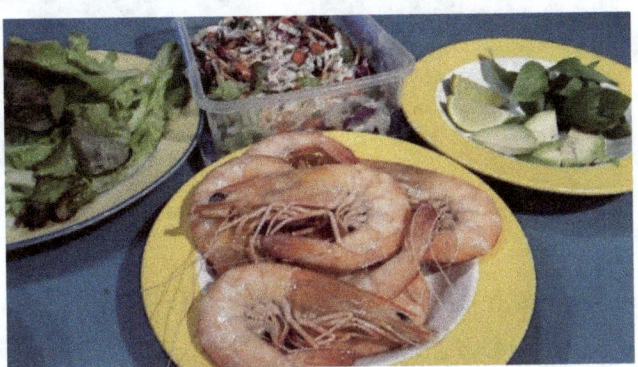

Figure 9: Fresh prawns and salad

- PRAWNS are 80% protein, with only 70calories per 100g; loads of B vitamins to support the nervous system; calcium and iron for the blood; and selenium for the immune system and thyroid health. Wild-caught prawns feed on small ocean creatures which makes them high in omega-3s and deliciously sweet, but they can be difficult to find. Farmed prawns are more readily available in supermarkets, but try to avoid imported prawns. Only buy prawns in their shells, as they have more flavour and are generally better quality.

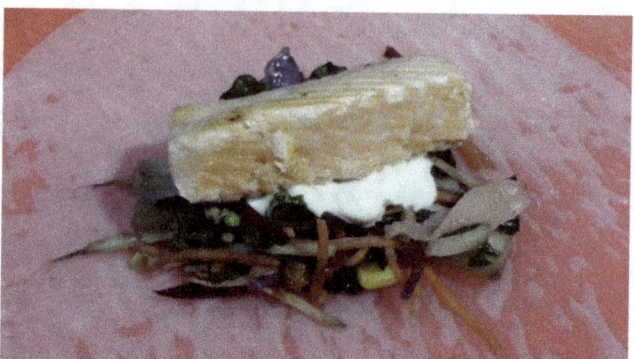

Figure 10: Rice paper roll with seared salmon fillet

- SALMON is a source of protein, omega-3s, vitamins B3, B12 and D, and phosphorus, but much higher in calories than tuna. I do like the flavour of wild-caught tinned Alaskan Red Salmon, much better than the cheaper pink salmon varieties, but I think tuna is a better filling for rice paper rolls, and half the price. You might enjoy the occasional fresh salmon fillet, pan-seared, but salmon has more calories than tuna, so make it a small serve.

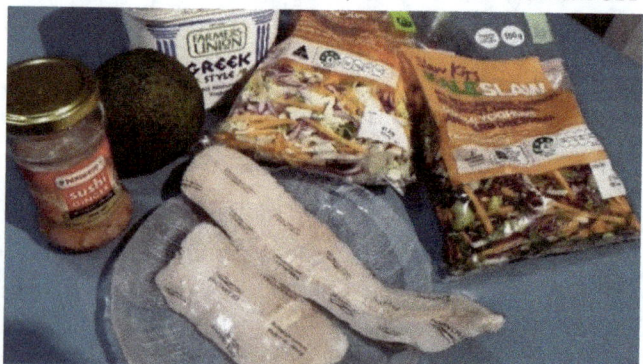

Figure 11: Frozen Hoki fillets, individually wrapped

- Individually wrapped frozen portions of WHITE FISH fillets, such as Hoki, make for a tasty and low-calorie dinner. Cook gently in a pan, as often as you like instead of tuna.

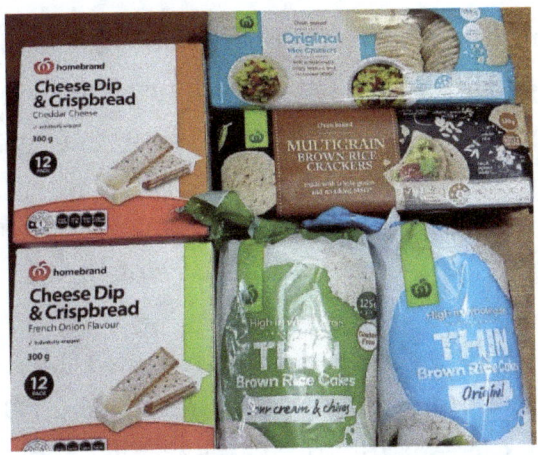

For something sweet or creamy, try one of these:
- A serving of fruit (check the list), with a good dollop of full-fat Greek-style yoghurt, or
- Blend half a serve of a chocolate or latte-flavoured diet powder with soy milk and ice cubes. Do NOT add bananas. On a hot summer's day, this can be a satisfying alternative to ice-cream, and it's full of vitamins and minerals too.

Smart snacks are a secret weapon. Arm yourself with a selection of well-chosen snack foods to give you that hit of sweet, savoury, salty, or sour. Preparation and planning are key to success.

We are all unique, and our mouths can be fussy eaters. But after a time, after eating more nutritious food, your mouth will develop a more discerning palate. You will become more aware of subtle flavours in your food, and your mouth will not be so lonely.

To lose weight, we need to consume fewer calories, so make every calorie count. Don't squander calories on foods that fail to give you (1) nutrition and (2) pleasure. Be fussy. Spend your money on quality produce, which does not have to be expensive. All snacks should be limited to between 150-250 calories each. Here are a few examples to use as a guide (details in the LET'S GO SHOPPING chapter):

- 99 cals = single serve of Woolworths Cheddar Cheese Snack, individual pantry packs of cheddar cheese with crackers
- 170 cals = 35g pitted sour bottled Morello Cherries (26cals) topped with 150g Greek yoghurt (140cals)
- 180 cals = 3x thin rice cakes (99cals), topped with 100g cottage cheese (80cals)
- 233 cals = 1x 110g tin of sardines
- 240 cals = 1x 25g row of rice crackers (104cals) dipped into 150g Greek yoghurt (140cals)

Friendly fluids

- Apple cider vinegar in cold water. This is what you drink each morning. The acidity changes the enzyme in your mouth, to stop you wanting carbohydrates.
- Another morning staple is Nature's Cuppa organic chai spiced tea (black tea bags, spiced with a combination of cinnamon, cardamon, ginger, cloves, black pepper, and pure vanilla bean). This tea has a warm spicy flavour and 'appetite suppressing' effect on the mouth. But from lunchtime onward, do not drink anything containing caffeine.

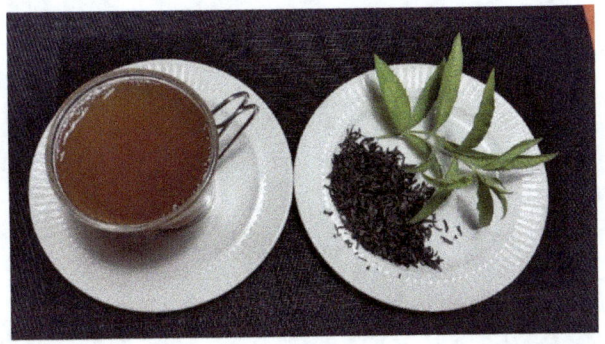

- Caffeine-free herbal infusions are excellent relaxers after dinner, especially a hot cup of camomile.
- Caffeine-free coffee substitutes are good to have on hand at night if your mouth is wanting a coffee or hot chocolate. Add soy milk for creaminess, and add a spoon of Avalanche sugar-free chocolate powder for a mocha flavour. (check the LET'S GO SHOPPING chapter for product details)
- And of course, don't forget to drink at least 3 or 4 big glasses of WATER every day. It keeps your cells hydrated, your digestion active, and your brain alert.

Smart snacks can satisfy your 'lonely' mouth

Chapter 15: Hunger Hero RECIPES

"Give a hungry person a fish, and they'll eat for a day. Teach them to fish, and they'll have the skills to eat for a lifetime."

This is where the HUNGER HERO DIET comes into its own. We have taken a sustainable approach. Instead of simply explaining the diet or handing you prepared meals, we have provided information so you can learn the fundamentals of nutritional biochemistry, neuroscience, and psychology. This is the equivalent of 'teaching you how to fish'.

This book provides you with the knowledge and skills to advance beyond the basic rules once you have lost a chunk of weight, to create your own lifestyle plan into the future. Think of it as a template, giving you the basic form and structure upon which you can build something that fits your personal preferences and lifestyle.

But you must learn to walk before you can run, so here is a chapter filled with recipes to get you started. Again, we have taken a practical approach with the recipes, making them easy to prepare, whether you're standing at the kitchen bench or sitting down for comfort. Even if you think you can't cook, you can make these easy recipes. And, we intentionally made everything suitable for ONE PERSON, as many of us live alone these days, or have to make separate meals for other family members. We have tried to make it as easy as possible, so EVERYONE has an equal opportunity to access an affordable weight loss solution.

This chapter shows how a few simple ingredients can be used in a multitude of ways. We start with basic recipes, and show you how to build upon these to create other dishes. And once you see how easy it is, you will only be limited by your imagination.

How to fold RICE PAPERS

For the first few weeks, you will be eating rice paper rolls for most meals, so you need to know how to make them.

Method

1. Place all ingredients and utensils on a clean kitchen bench.
2. If you can, sit down at the kitchen bench, as this helps the process.
3. Set aside THREE sheets of rice paper (dinner plate size)
4. Place a large flat plate or tray on the bench. Must be large enough to allow for a sheet of rice paper to be submerged in water.

5. Add a little room temperature tap water to the large plate. (Do not use warm water of the rice paper will soften too quickly.)
6. Submerge one sheet of rice paper in the water. Give it a little poke with your finger to keep it under water. After a few seconds, before it goes limp, take it out of the water and lay it flat on the kitchen bench, or on a plastic cutting board.
7. Quickly build the filling on one side of the wet wrapper, before it becomes too limp to manage. Add the wet ingredients first, and finish with the dry salad – it acts as a protective cover and makes it less messy to roll up.
8. Once you have all your filling arranged on the rice paper, carefully lift the nearest edge and fold over to cover the filling. By starting at the front, you can then fold the sides, and finish by rolling it to the other end. You should have a neat parcel.
9. REPEAT until you have THREE RICE PAPER ROLLS arranged neatly on a small plate. Take a quick pic of your finished creation.

HINT: Wet rice paper quickly softens to become limp and sticky, so don't be surprised if your first few attempts look untidy. If you make a mess, wrap the whole thing in a large lettuce leaf to hold it together. The trick is to get the filling done quickly, before the rice paper becomes too soft and sticky, so just make one roll at a time.

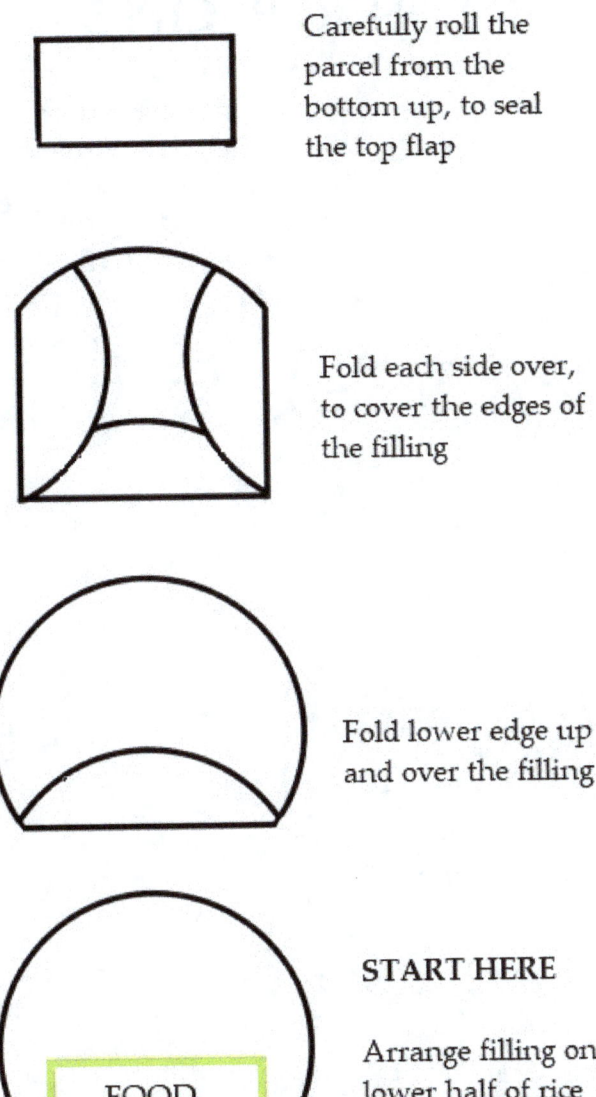

Carefully roll the parcel from the bottom up, to seal the top flap

Fold each side over, to cover the edges of the filling

Fold lower edge up and over the filling

START HERE

Arrange filling on lower half of rice paper

FOOD

LUNCH RECIPES

Recipe: Tinned TUNA rice paper rolls

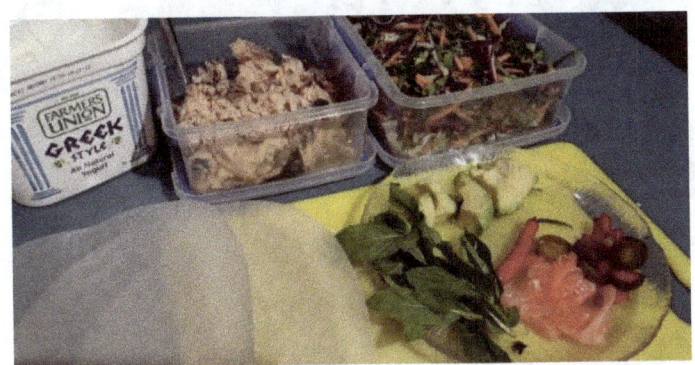

To make THREE rice paper rolls (one portion), you will need:
- 3 large circles of dried rice paper (10 to a pack)
- 200g tinned tuna in springwater
- 3 dessert spoons of natural full-fat Greek-style yoghurt
- 3 dessert spoons of diced fresh herbs, such as dill, coriander, fennel fronds, Thai basil, or Vietnamese mint. (Avoid European parsley and basil, as they do not suit the Asian flavour profile of this dish.)
- About a cup of dry mixed coleslaw salad (without dressing), just enough so you can still roll the wrapper over the filling. Most salads contain shredded cabbage, carrot, celery, and onion.
- 6 strips of Pandaroo Japanese sweet pickled pink sushi ginger (optional)
- A touch of something spicy, such as a teaspoon of sambal oelek (minced chili) or a few slices of pickled jalapenos (optional).
- ¼ ripe avocado (optional, but not every day)

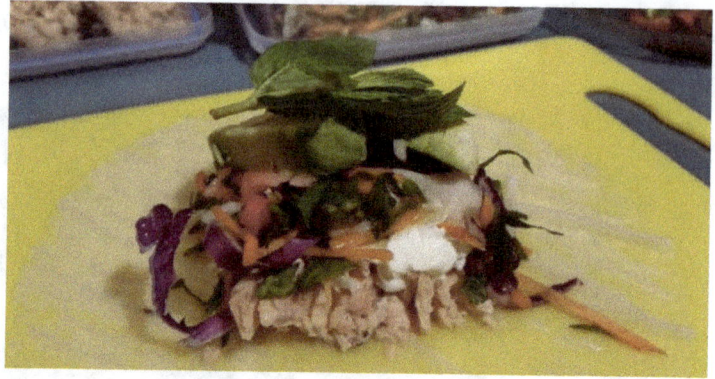

Method

- Get everything out and onto the kitchen bench.
- Sit down at the kitchen bench, to help you stay focussed.

- Follow the recipe HOW TO FOLD RICE PAPERS
- REPEAT until you have THREE RICE PAPER ROLLS arranged neatly on a small plate. Take a quick pic of your finished creation.

HINT: Most pre-packaged salads and slaws contain 'salad toppers' – sachets of salad dressing and fried noodles. These are extra calories without nutritional value. Toss them in the bin. Store leftover salads in plastic storage containers and return to fridge until needed. Do not mix salads with different 'use by' dates.

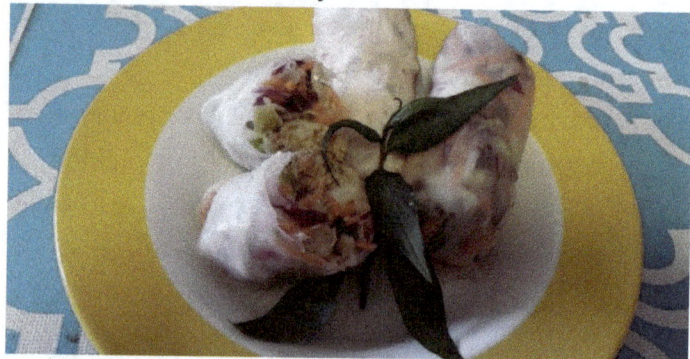

Recipe: PRAWN rice paper rolls

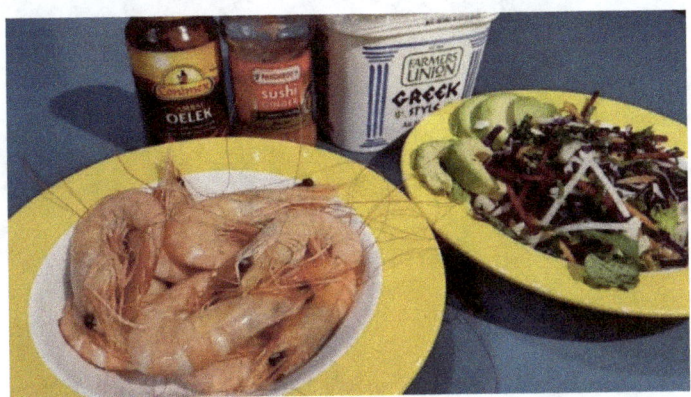

To make THREE rice paper rolls (one portion), you will need:
- 3 large circles of dried rice paper (10 to a pack)
- 6 medium/large size prawns (in their shells)
- 3 dessert spoons of natural full-fat Greek-style yoghurt
- 3 dessert spoons of diced fresh herbs, such as dill, coriander, fennel fronds, Thai basil, or Vietnamese mint. (Avoid European parsley and basil, as they do not suit the Asian flavour profile of this dish.)
- About a cup of dry mixed coleslaw salad (without dressing), just enough so you can still roll the wrapper over the filling. Most salads contain shredded cabbage, carrot, celery, and onion.
- 6 strips of Pandaroo Japanese sweet pickled pink sushi ginger (optional)
- A touch of something spicy, such as a teaspoon of sambal oelek (minced chili) or a few slices of pickled jalapenos (optional).
- ¼ ripe avocado (optional, but not every day)

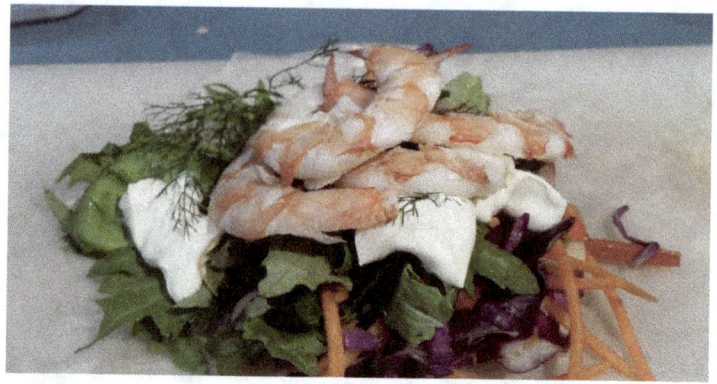

Method

- Get everything out and onto the kitchen bench.
- Sit down at the kitchen bench, to help you stay focussed.

- Peel and devein just enough prawns for this meal. Grab the head and firmly remove it from the body. Remove remaining shell, legs, and tail. To de-vein, run a sharp knife down the spine of the prawn, to reveal the intestine. In farmed prawns, this may be a thin white thread because they haven't eaten recently. In wild-caught prawns, this is usually a thick black thread because they have been feeding. Whatever you see, remove it. Rinse in a little water or white vinegar if any dark bits remain. If you're not sure, there are lots of videos on the internet, if you search for them. **TIP**: Store the discarded shells in a covered bowl in the fridge or freezer until you're ready to throw them out.
- Follow the recipe HOW TO FOLD RICE PAPERS
- REPEAT until you have THREE RICE PAPER ROLLS arranged neatly on a small plate. Take a quick pic of your finished creation.

HINT: Most pre-packaged salads and slaws contain 'salad toppers' – sachets of salad dressing and fried noodles. These are extra calories without nutritional value. Toss them in the bin. Store leftover salads in plastic storage containers and return to fridge until needed. Do not mix salads with different 'use by' dates.

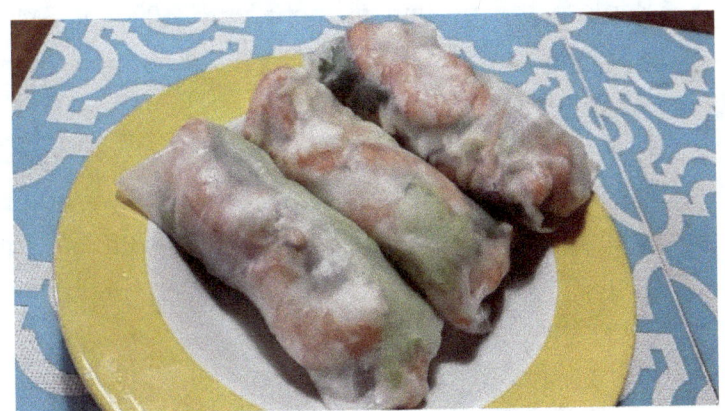

LUNCH VARIATIONS

Experiment with different combinations of herbs and salad vegetables.

- Add fresh sprouts for a crunchy textural change.
- Add ¼ ripe avocado for a smooth and silky texture, but not every day.
- Replace the protein element with 100g of SMOKED SALMON or SMOKED TROUT, but no more than once a week.
- If you wish, slices of flavoured tofu can be used as a low-calorie protein substitute, but not too often. You don't want to miss out on the crucial health benefits, for your mind and body, of eating good quality seafood every day.
- Once a month, if you miss your deli meats, replace the protein element with 100g of best quality HAM OFF THE BONE. Change the condiments in your rice paper rolls to suit the ham, with a little creamed horseradish, Dijon mustard, mustard pickles, or mayonnaise. Maybe use lettuce leaves instead of coleslaw salad mix as your vegetable element.
- Once or twice a week, turn leftover salad vegetables or leafy greens into a delicious one-pan wonder of POACHED EGGS with STEAMED VEGES (see recipe). Perfect for lunch or dinner, or a weekend brunch.
- MEDITERRANEAN TOMATO SALAD with tinned tuna or feta cheese (see recipe). This dish is an alternative lunch or dinner meal. To make it a low-calorie afternoon snack, omit the tuna and feta cheese.

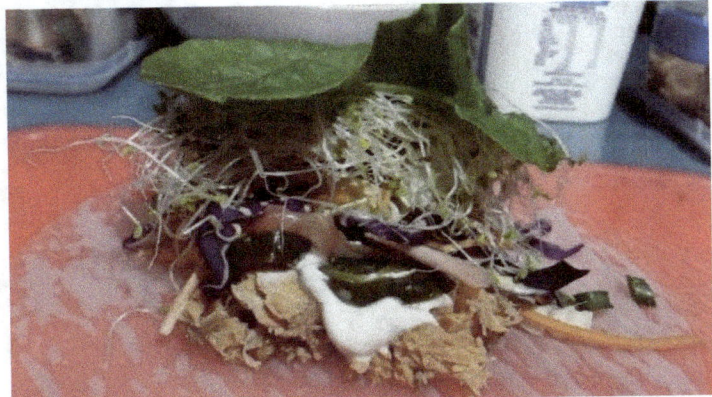
Figure 14: Rice paper rolls with tinned tuna and sprouts

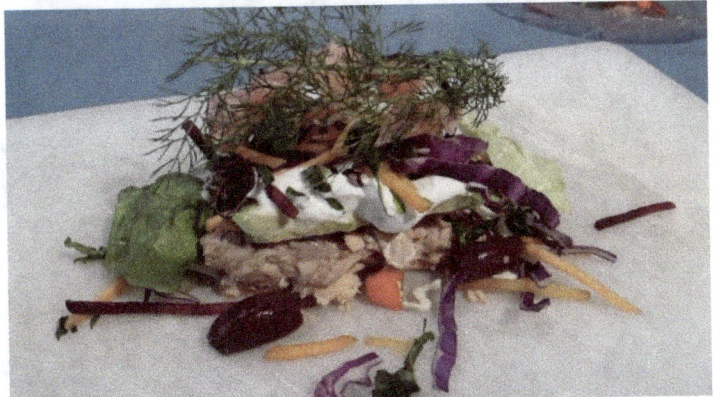
Figure 15: Rice paper rolls with tinned tuna and black olives

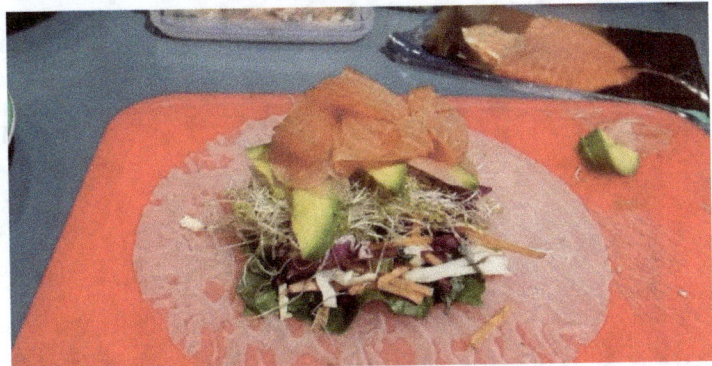
Figure 16: Rice paper rolls with smoked salmon and avocado

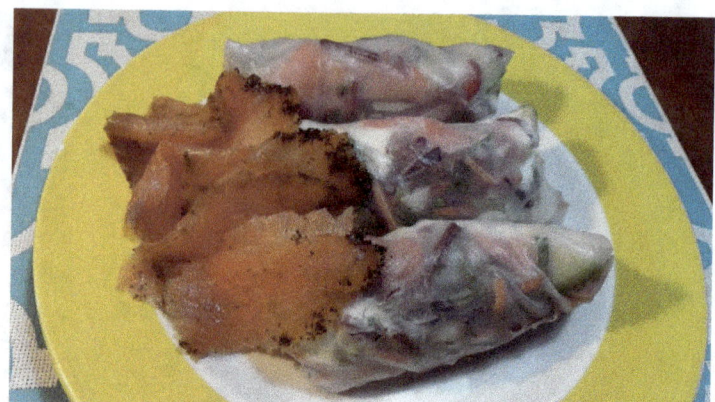

Figure 17: Rice paper rolls with smoked trout and avocado

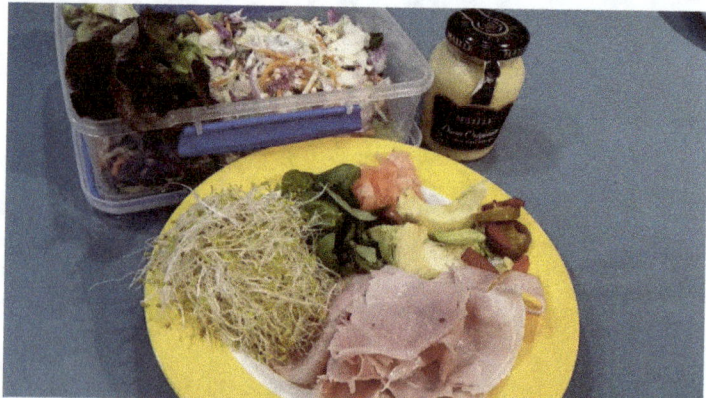

Figure 18: Making rice paper rolls with shaved ham and Dijon

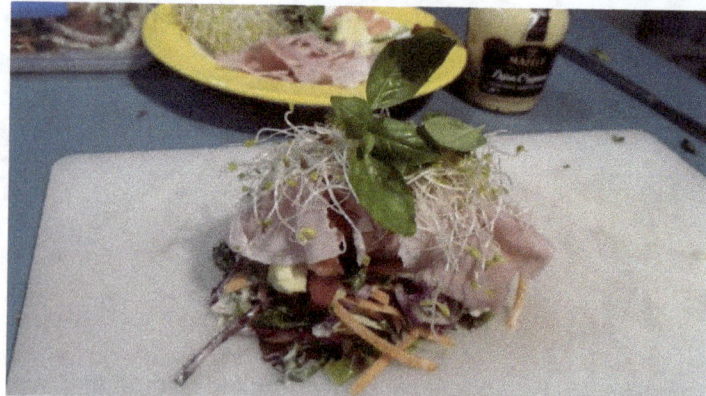

Figure 19: Rice paper rolls with shaved ham, Dijon mustard, basil

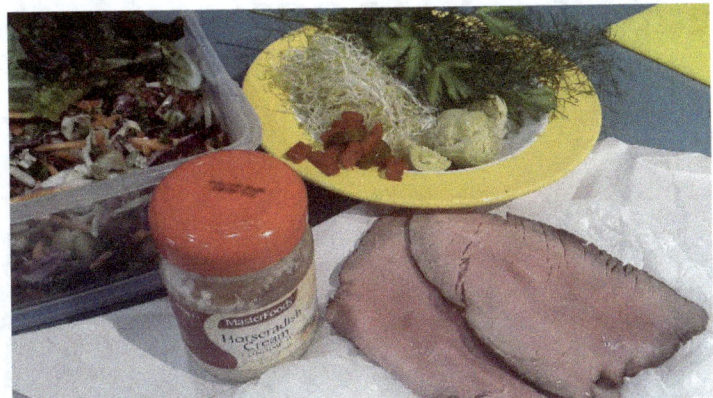

Figure 20: Making rice paper rolls with corned beef and horseradish cream

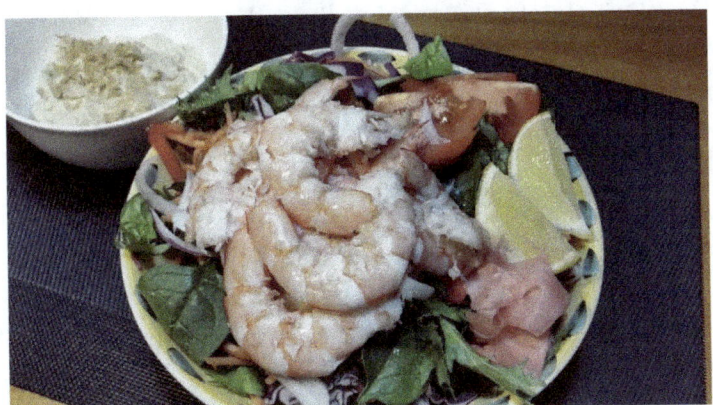

Figure 21: Prawn salad bowl

Recipe: Poached EGGS & braised veg

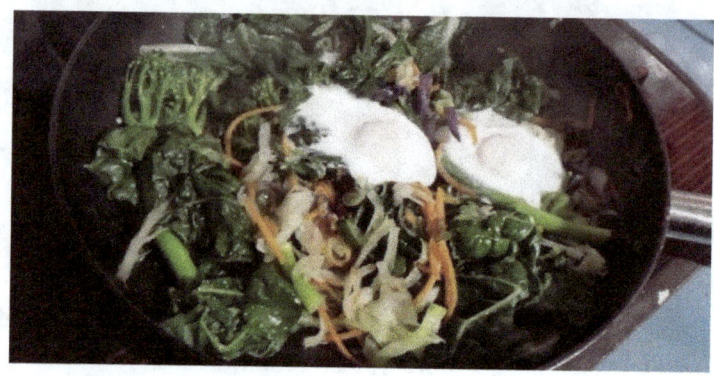

- Non-stick pan with a lid
- Drizzle of extra virgin olive oil
- 2 cups leftover salad veges or leafy greens
- 2 large free-range eggs
- Salt, cracked pepper
- Dollop of Greek yoghurt and squeeze of lemon

Method

- Heat pan on high, add oil
- Add veges, and stir for a couple of minutes until they soften
- Crack in 2 whole eggs right on top of the veges
- Season with salt and cracked pepper
- Turn the heat down to medium, and cover with a lid.
- When the tops of the eggs turn white, the eggs are cooked but still runny. Turn off the heat.
- Serve as poached eggs, OR
- Using a large spatula, gently flip the mixture over for a few seconds to crisp the top side, to create a VEG OMELETTE. Serve with yoghurt and lemon juice.

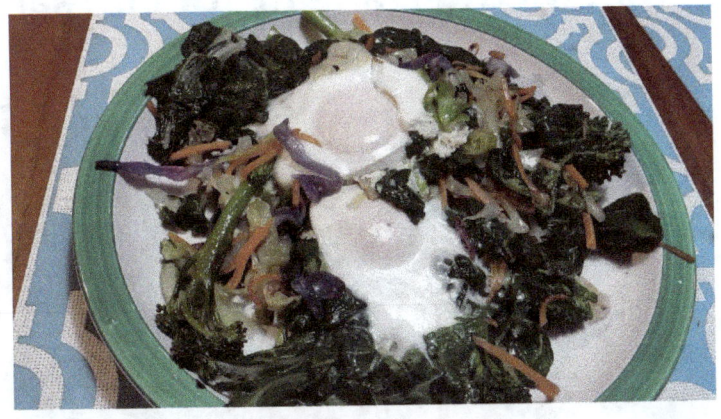

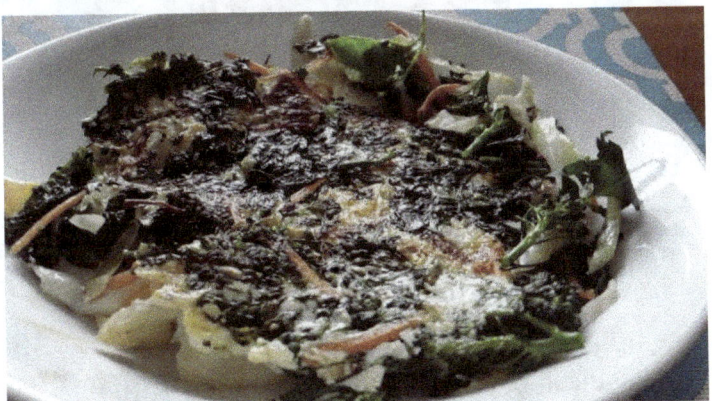

Figure 22: Flipped in the pan to create a vegetable omelette

Recipe: Mediterranean tomato salad

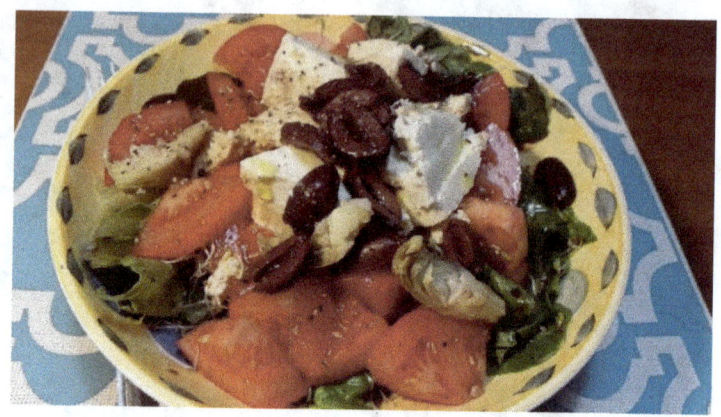

- 200g of chunky tuna OR 80g feta cheese
- A few lettuce leaves, any variety
- 1 ripe red tomato, diced
- 1-2 artichoke halves, bottled or canned, sliced (optional)
- Fresh basil or dill
- A few black olives (optional)
- A splash of Balsamic vinegar
- A drizzle of extra virgin olive oil
- Salt and cracked pepper

Method
- Place all ingredients in a bowl
- Drizzle with a little extra virgin olive oil and Balsamic vinegar (or apple cider vinegar, or lemon juice)
- Season with salt and cracked pepper

AFTERNOON SNACKS

The basic afternoon snack is 3 thin rice cakes spread with cottage cheese. It's tangy and crunchy, and sure to become a favourite dish, but sometimes you will want to jazz it up.

- Add something a little zesty but low calorie, such as sliced tomato, beetroot, cucumber, jalapenos, or olives.
- Add 50g SMOKED SALMON to your usual rice cakes and cottage cheese, top with a little coriander or dill.

VARIATIONS (instead of rice cakes)

- Snack on ½ tin of dolmades
- Snack on ¼ packet of Macro Honey Soy Tofu, or Satay Tofu (less than 100cals), straight from the fridge
- Indulge with 6 fresh oysters in their shell (less than 100cals)
- Enjoy a small bowl of MEDITERRANEAN TOMATO SALAD (see lunch **RECIPE**, but without the feta cheese or tuna)

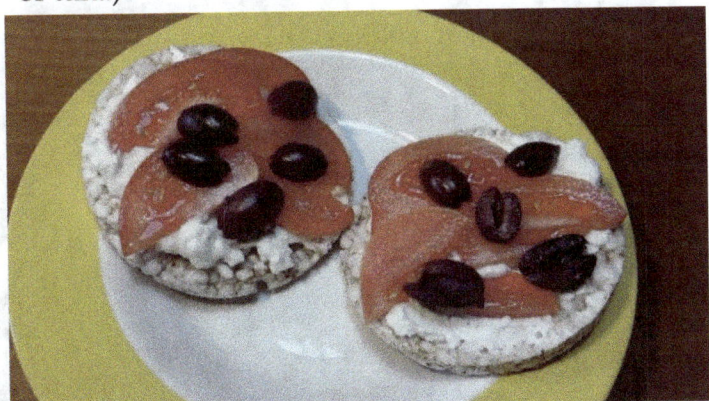

Figure 23: Rice cakes, cottage cheese, tomato and black olives

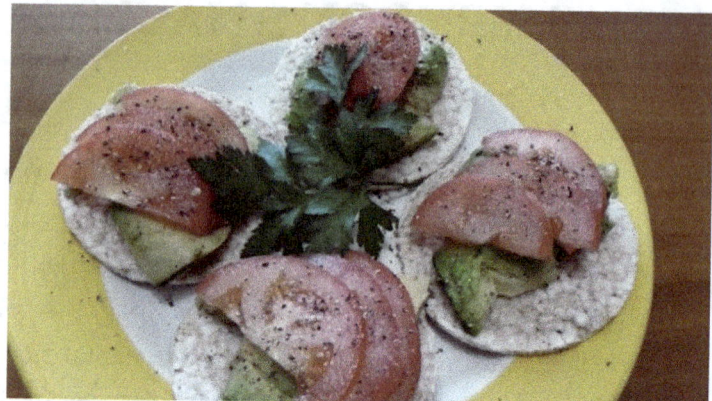

Figure 24: Rice cakes with avocado and sliced tomato

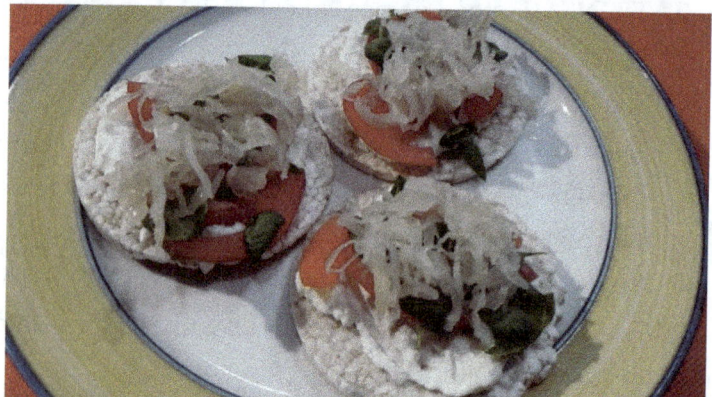

Figure 25: Rice cakes, cottage cheese, tomato, and sauerkraut

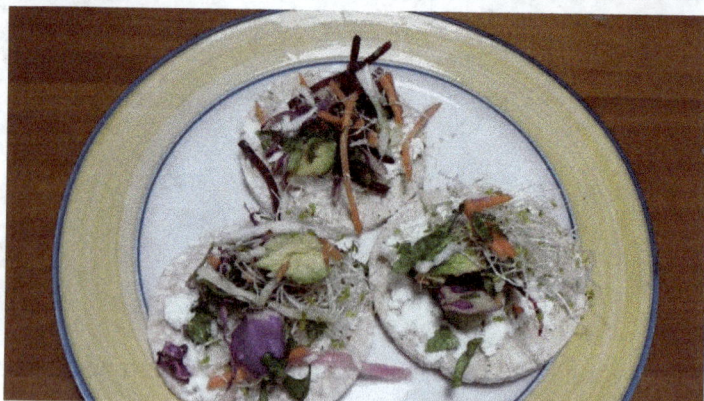

Figure 26: Rice cakes with cottage cheese, avo cado, salad

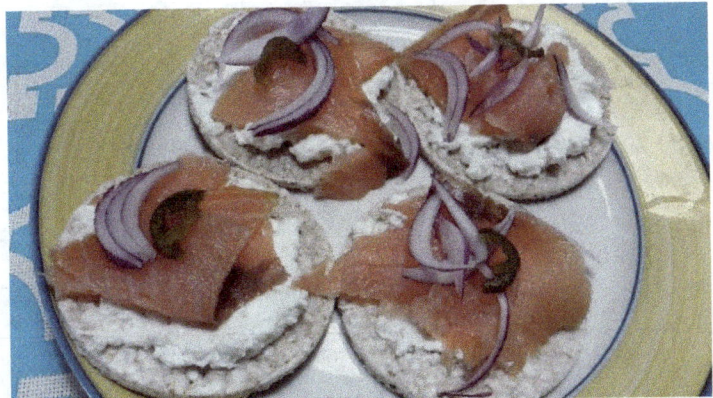

Figure 27: Rice cakes, cottage cheese, smoked salmon, onion

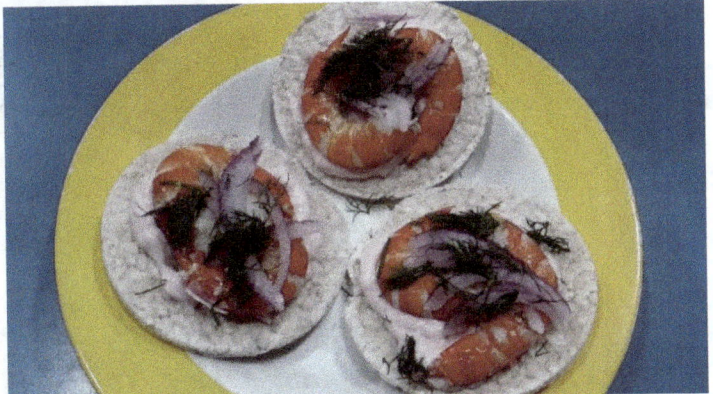

Figure 28: Rice cakes with cottage cheese, prawns, onion, dill

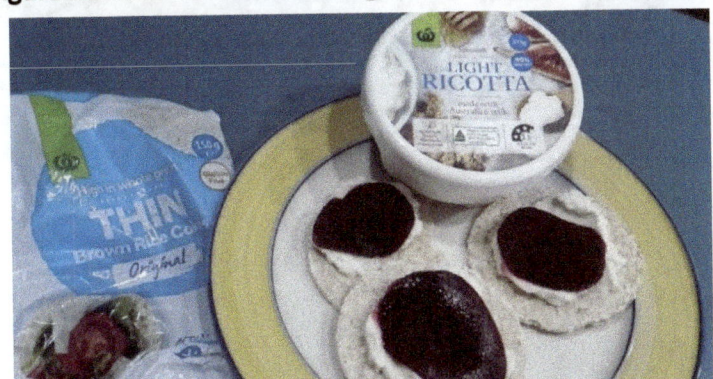

Figure 29: Rice cakes with ricotta cheese and tinned beetroot

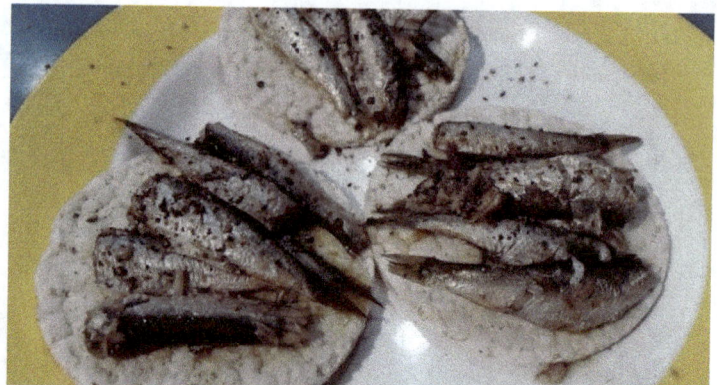

Figure 30: Rice cakes with tinned sardines, salt, cracked pepper

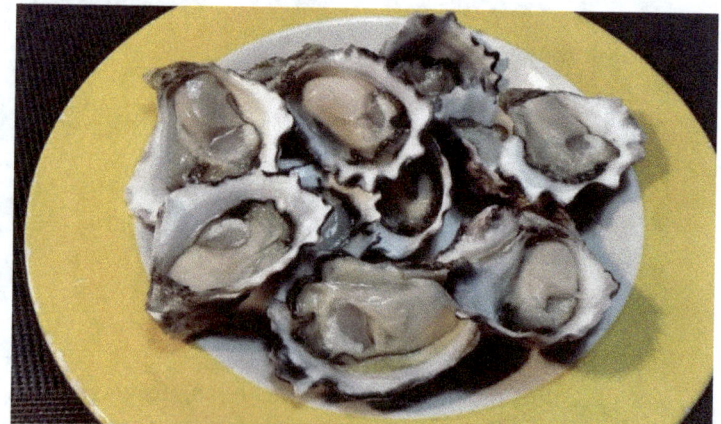

Figure 31: Freshly shucked oysters with lemon juice

DINNER RECIPES

Recipe: Pan-seared TUNA STEAK

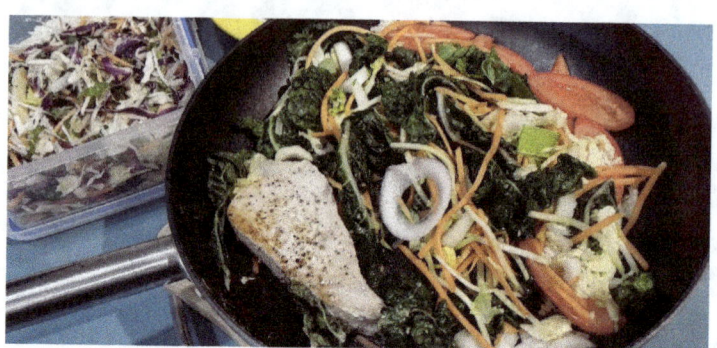

These hot and juicy slices of freshly cooked tuna steak make for a delicious main ingredient for your evening meal – in rice paper rolls, or in one of the many noodle bowl recipes.

If you like, add a small serve of broccoli (or other vegetables) to the same pan and cook them together.

- Small non-stick pan
- Drizzle of extra virgin olive oil
- 1 thawed TUNA steak
- Salt, cracked pepper
- 1 small head of broccoli, or a bunch of other greens (optional)
- Squeeze of lemon juice (optional)

Method

- Heat pan on high, add a drizzle of oil
- Add TUNA STEAK to hot pan
- Add sliced BROCCOLI to pan (if desired)
- Cook for a couple of minutes, giving the underside of the tuna a chance to get brown and a little crusty
- Season with salt and cracked pepper
- Flip the tuna steak and toss broccoli

- Leave to cook for another minute or so. But if using broccoli, cover pan with a lid so steam can cook the thick stalks.
- Remove pan from heat
- Remove tuna steak from pan and slice into thick strips.

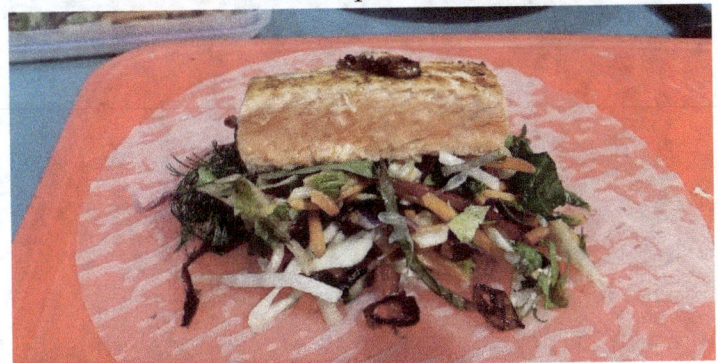

TIP: The tuna should be medium-rare, with a thin pink line through the centre of the steak. If you cook it longer, it can become a little dry and tough. But if you do want to cook it a bit more, leave the steak in the pan for a minute or so after turning off the heat. The residual heat will cook it further. Serve the cooked veges with a squeeze of lemon juice, as a side dish to the rice paper rolls, or in a noodle dish.

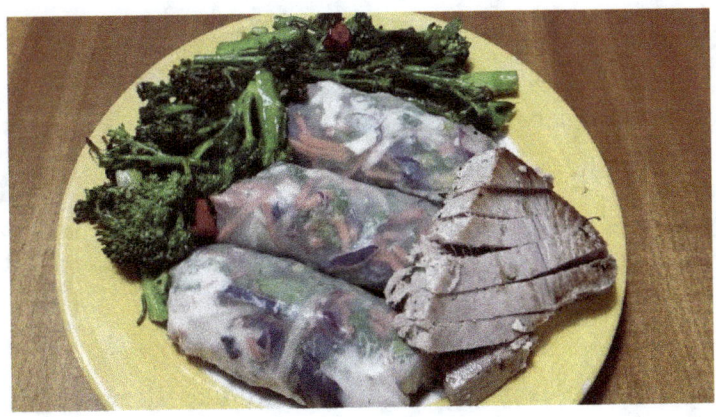

Recipe: Pan-fried thin WHITE FISH

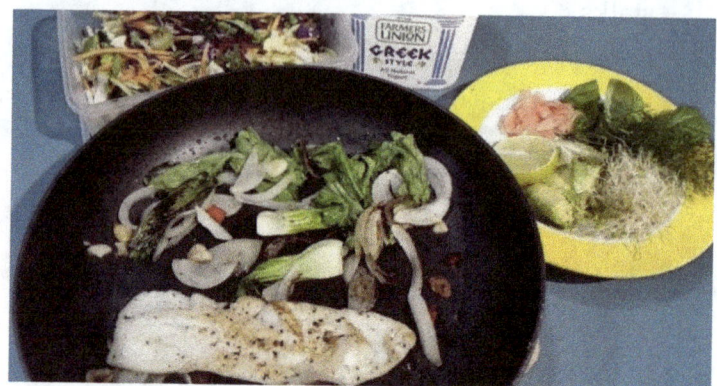

This recipe is suitable for thin fillets of white fish such as New Zealand Hoki, especially when cooked with leafy Asian greens, as they have the same cooking time.

- Small non-stick pan
- Drizzle of extra virgin olive oil
- 1 or 2 fillets of thawed WHITE FISH (Hoki)
- Salt, cracked pepper
- 1 small baby bok choy, or other leafy greens (optional)
- Squeeze of lemon juice (optional)

Method

- Heat pan on high, add a drizzle of oil
- Add fish fillet to pan
- Add leafy greens to pan (if desired)
- Cook for a couple of minutes
- Season with salt and cracked pepper
- When the edges of the fish fillet start to turn white, flip the fillet and toss the vegetables
- Cook for another minute or so

TIP: If cooking a thicker fish like Barramundi, or a thicker vegetable like broccoli, cover pan with a lid for

a few minutes so the steam can finish the cooking. You can add a spoonful of water to help the process.
- Remove pan from heat. Remove fish and allow to cool a little before making rice paper rolls. If the fish is too warm, the rice paper will go soft too quickly.
- Construct your RICE PAPER ROLLS with salad, in the usual manner. Serve with warm Asian greens on the side, with a lemon wedge.

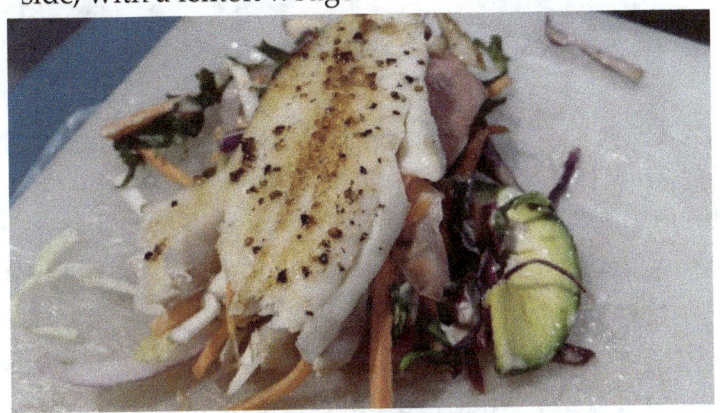

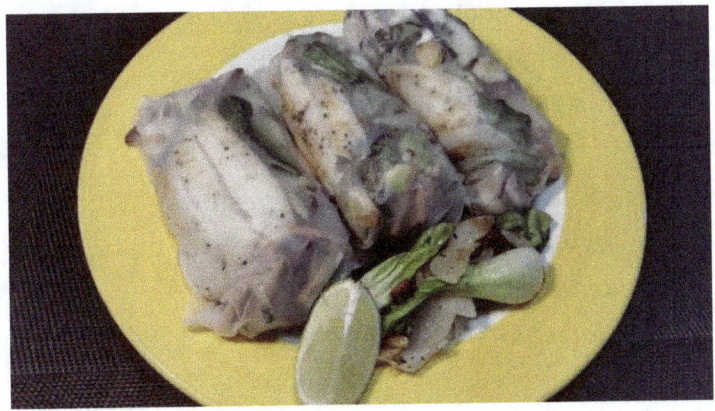

Recipe: Crispy skin SALMON fillet

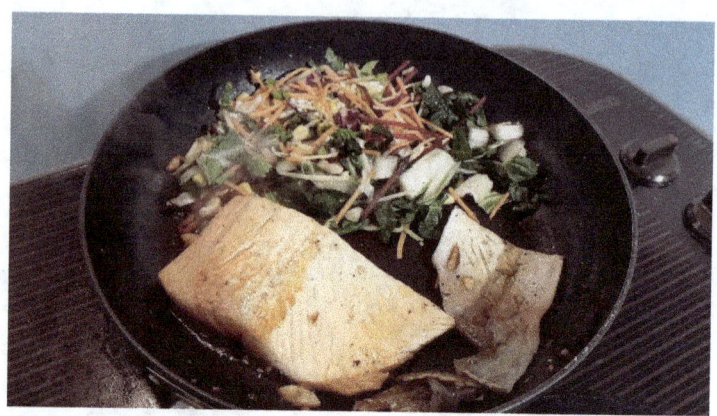

This recipe explains how to cook a fresh Tasmanian salmon fillet, with the skin on. Salmon has a distinctly rich flavour, and the crispy skin makes for an occasional treat. The correct way to cook a salmon fillet is medium-rare, when the centre is warm but still pink – but you can cook it all the way through if that's what you prefer. (If making rice paper rolls, use a smaller fillet.)

- Small non-stick pan
- Drizzle of extra virgin olive oil
- 1 small SALMON FILLET, with skin on
- Salt, cracked pepper
- A handful of dry coleslaw vegetables
- 1 large leaf of silverbeet, chopped, or other leafy greens
- Squeeze of lemon juice
- Dollop of Greek yoghurt

Method

Step 1

- Heat pan on high, add drizzle of oil , salt, cracked pepper
- Add fish fillet to pan, SKIN SIDE DOWN

- Add vegetables
- Allow the fish to cook until the skin has browned and become crispy

Step 2
- Drizzle a little oil over the fish, then flip it over
- Using utensils, carefully peel the skin from the fish
- Place the skin in the pan, crispy side up – allowing the fatty side to cook. DO NOT COVER THE PAN
- Leave everything to cook for another minute or so

Step 3
- Season with salt and cracked pepper again
- Remove pan from heat
- Transfer vegetables and fish to a bowl. Arrange crispy skin on top.
- Serve with squeeze of lemon juice and a dollop of natural yoghurt.

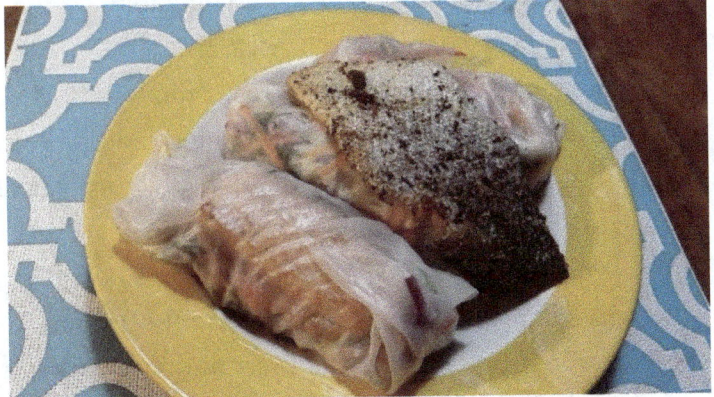

HINT: If making rice paper rolls, allow everything to cool a little before doing so. If the filling is too warm, the rice paper will go soft too quickly and make it hard to roll. Alternatively, cook the salmon without vegetables, and use salad in your RICE PAPER ROLLS.

DINNER VARIATIONS

All types of seafood lend themselves to being cooked gently in a pan with mixed vegetables or served with a salad and tasty dressing.

Or for a change of pace on colder nights, drop a few slices of raw fish and a serve of Asian greens into a bowl of steaming stock broth for a quick and tasty soup.

The same basic ingredients can become so many different dishes – rice paper rolls, salads, soups, or one-pan wonders. Once you get the basics, you are only limited by your imagination.

- Rice paper rolls with pan-fried WHITE FISH (Hoki) and broccoli
- Pan-fried WHITE FISH (Hoki) and red capsicum
- Sauteed MARINARA MIX and vegetables
- Oven-baked 'pizza-style' MUSHROOM CAPS with passata sauce, European herbs, onion, cottage cheese (better if you remove the stalks before adding topping)
- Barbequed MUSHROOM CAPS with European herbs, ricotta cheese, shaved ham
- If you want to lose weight, you won't be eating meat more than once a month. Pork is the preferred meat across Asia, so that is what I recommend. Pork is a good fit with the Asian-inspired HUNGER HERO menu, and it is usually much cheaper than beef or lamb. The serving size for pork is just under 200g, which is the usual size of a single pork scotch fillet steak from the supermarket. Try a PAN-FRIED PORK SCOTCH FILLET (see **RECIPE**).

If you cannot eat pork, for any reason, you can forego the occasional steak or choose a different type of meat in a smaller portion size. Avoid minced meat, as it has much more saturated fat than a piece of good quality steak, and none of the chemical preservatives.

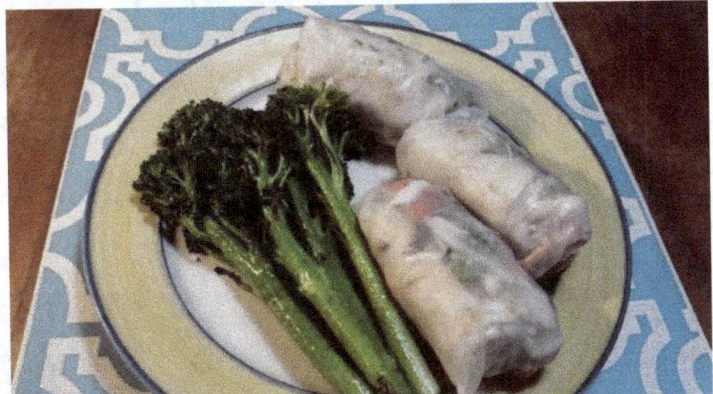

Figure 32: Rice paper rolls with white fish (Hoki) and broccoli

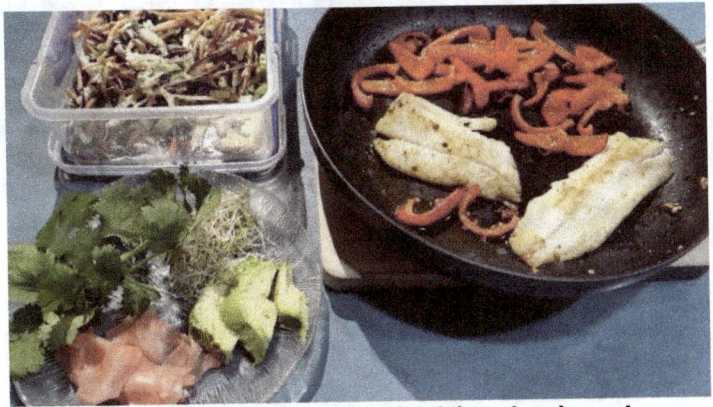

Figure 33: Pan-fried white fish (Hoki) and red capsicum

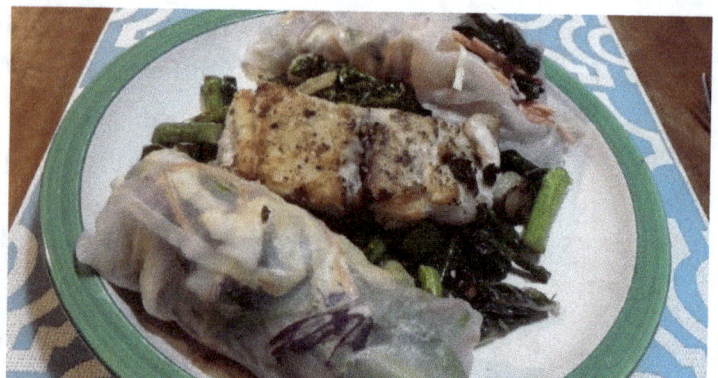
Figure 34: Rice paper rolls with pan-fried white fish (Barramundi)

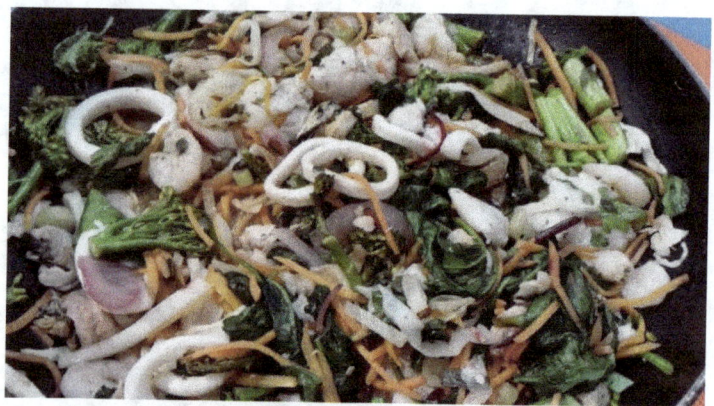
Figure 35: Sauteed 'marinara mix' and vegetables

Recipe: Thick WHITE FISH, braised veg

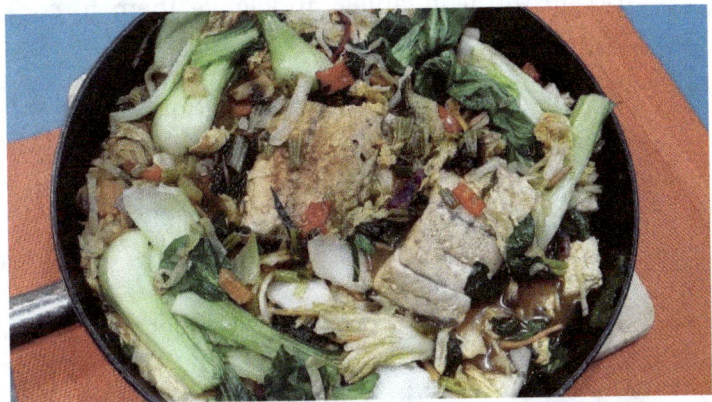

This is suitable for cooking thick fillets like Barramundi.

- Medium non-stick pan, with a lid
- Drizzle of extra virgin olive oil
- 1 fillet of Barramundi, or other thick white fish, skin off
- 2 cups of dry coleslaw mix
- 1 small baby bok choy, or other leafy greens
- 1 small chili, or a teaspoon of Sambal Oelek chili paste
- A heaped teaspoon of vegetable stock powder
- 1 cup of boiling water
- Salt and cracked pepper
- Squeeze of lemon juice (optional)

Method

Step 1

- Heat pan on high, add a drizzle of oil
- Add fish fillet to pan
- Season with salt and cracked pepper
- Add chopped chili, or Sambal Oelek chili paste
- Cook for a couple of minutes
- Flip fish onto the other side, just for a few seconds, then remove from pan and set aside on a plate

Step 2

- Into empty pan, add another drizzle of oil
- Add all the vegetables, and leave them to cook for a minute in the oil
- Sprinkle the teaspoon of stock powder over the vegetables
- Pour a cup of hot water over the stock powder
- Give everything a light stir

Step 3

- Lay the partially cooked fish fillet on top of the vegetables

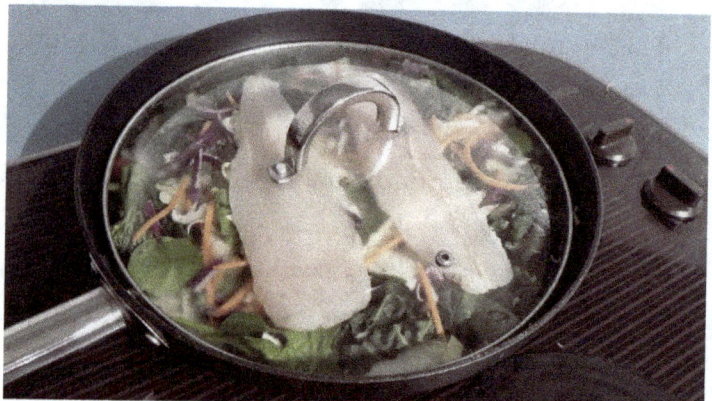

- Cover with a lid, and leave to cook for a couple of minutes. The steam will quickly cook through the thick fish while keeping it moist.
- Remove pan from heat. Transfer everything into a bowl.
- Serve with a squeeze of lemon juice. Adjust seasonings if desired.

Recipe: Pan-fried PORK scotch fillet

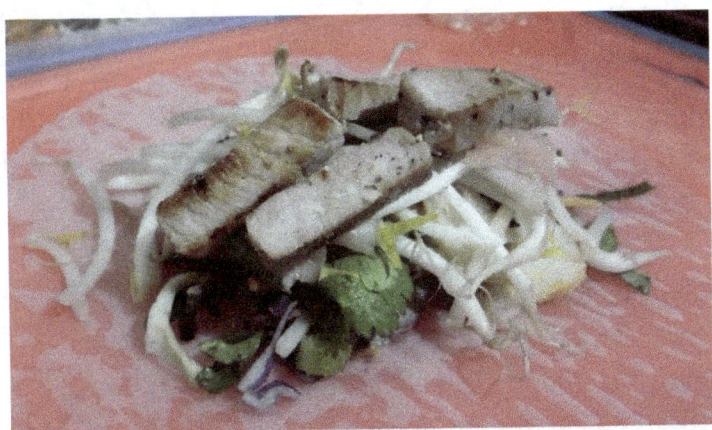

These hot and juicy slices of freshly cooked pork scotch fillet make for a delicious alternative to the pan-fried TUNA STEAKS, but limit them to once every couple of weeks if you want to lose weight.

- Non-stick pan, drizzle of extra virgin olive oil
- 1 x PORK scotch fillet steak, about 200g, at room temperature
- Salt and cracked pepper
- 1 small head of broccoli, sliced (optional)
- Squeeze of fresh lemon or lime juice (optional)

Method

- Heat pan on high, add oil
- Add PORK SCOTCH FILLET STEAK to pan
- Sear one side, then the other, as you do with the tuna steaks. But you need to cook the pork for a few minutes longer on both sides.
- When you flip the steak to cook the other side, add your veges, season with salt and pepper, and add another drizzle of olive oil.

- Cover with lid and steam for a couple of minutes until cooked.
- Take pan off heat, remove lid. Leave pork to rest for a minute.
- Transfer pork to a cutting board and cut into strips.
- If you cooked veges in the pan, serve them on the side of the plate with a squeeze of lemon juice.

HINTS: If making rice paper rolls with warm ingredients, be careful. Warm, food will make the rice paper go very limp, very quickly. Get them packed and rolled as fast as you can. But it's worth it. The warm filling is delicious.

Sometimes I thaw the frozen pork steak just enough to get the kitchen knife into it, then cut it into strips. I toss them into the heated pan with a little oil, salt and pepper, then brown all sides. This is quick and easy. Cooks in seconds.

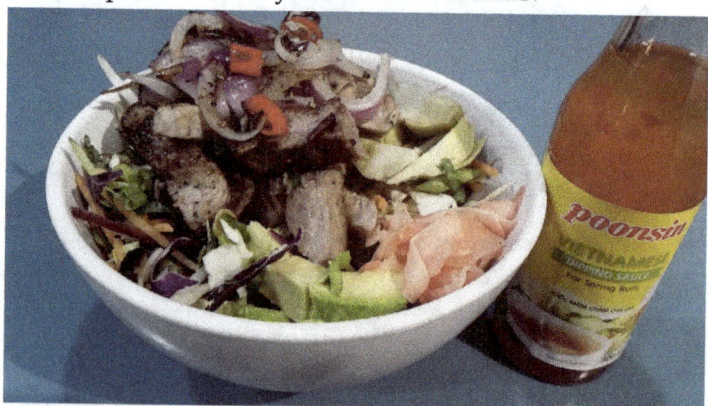

Figure 36: Pork scotch fillet with salad & Asian dressing

Recipe: Stuffed MUSHROOM CAPS

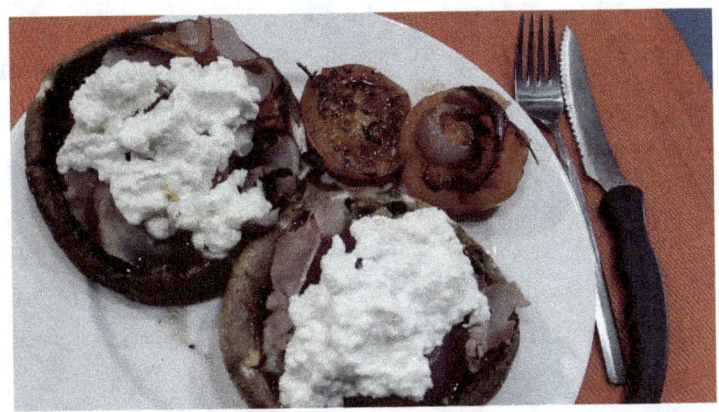

Baked or barbequed stuffed mushroom caps are delicious when freshly cooked, but leftovers are equally delicious as a cold snack the next day. The cooked stalks are yummy too! Store leftovers in a paper-lined plastic tub. They will keep in the fridge for a couple of days.

- 6-12 large fresh mushroom caps, brown or white
- A heated oven with baking tray and baking paper, OR
- BBQ grill
- a filling of your choice, with cottage cheese or ricotta
- plus, a slice of cheddar cheese (if desired)
- salt and cracked pepper

Method

- Pre-heat the cooking device – oven or BBQ
- Give mushrooms a gentle wipe with damp hands and kitchen paper. Do not wash them.
- Gently tear the stalks away from the caps, and put to one side.

- Arrange the mushroom caps on a flat surface. Add your preferred topping (see below for ideas). Season with salt, cracked pepper, herbs and spices.
- If grilling on a BBQ, transfer stuffed mushroom caps and the loose stalks to the grill and close the lid.
- If oven baking, transfer stuffed mushroom caps and the loose stalks to a shallow baking tray that has been covered in a sheet of baking paper. (The stalks make a tasty snack on their own, so don't throw them out.)
- Cook on high for approximately 20 minutes

TOPPINGS

- Pizza-style MUSHROOM CAPS – the filling has a splash of tomato passata, a chopped tomato, Italian dried herbs, onion rings, chili, and cottage cheese. This image shows mushroom stalks intact, with fresh rosemary, but you can use whatever you like. (Oven-baked or BBQ)
- MUSHROOM CAPS with ricotta cheese, fresh European herbs, and shaved smoked ham (Oven-baked or BBQ)
- MUSHROOM CAPS smeared with a little pesto sauce from a jar, topped with pimento-stuffed green olives, and cheese (cottage or ricotta), are delicious. Add a little shaved ham if you like. Use your imagination, and come up with some flavour sensations.

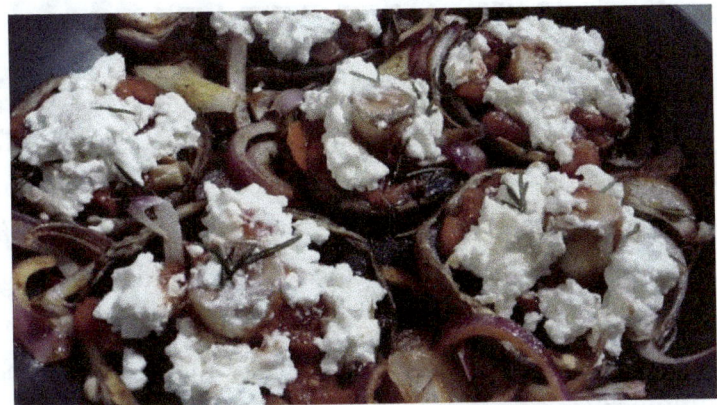
Figure 37: Pizza-style mushroom caps

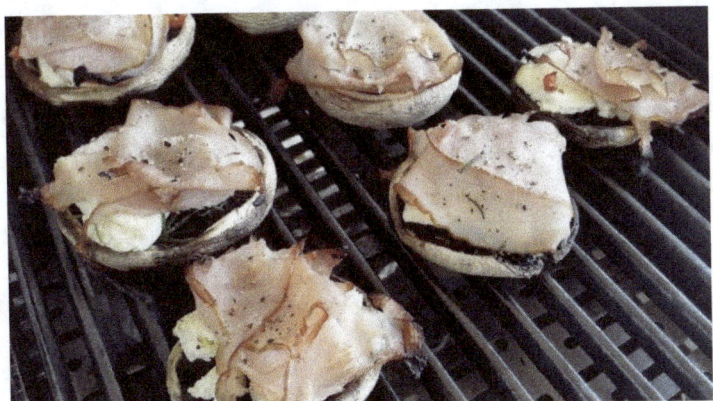
Figure 38: BBQ Mushroom caps with shaved ham and ricotta

Recipe: Grilled VEGETABLES

Grilled seasonal vegetables – glistening in olive oil, and sprinkled with fragrant European herbs – make a delicious side dish or snack, especially in the winter months. Cruciferous greens and root vegetables are equally tantalising – eggplant (aubergine), broccoli, carrots, beetroot, capsicum (bell peppers), tomatoes, broccolini, Brussels sprouts, sweet potato, cauliflower.

Think 'Italian antipasti'. Grab whatever vegetables and herbs are in season, cook up a storm. **Serve as accompaniments to your other dishes, or as tasty snacks with a squeeze of lemon juice and a dollop of Greek yoghurt.** Leftovers should keep in plastic containers in the fridge for a couple of weeks.

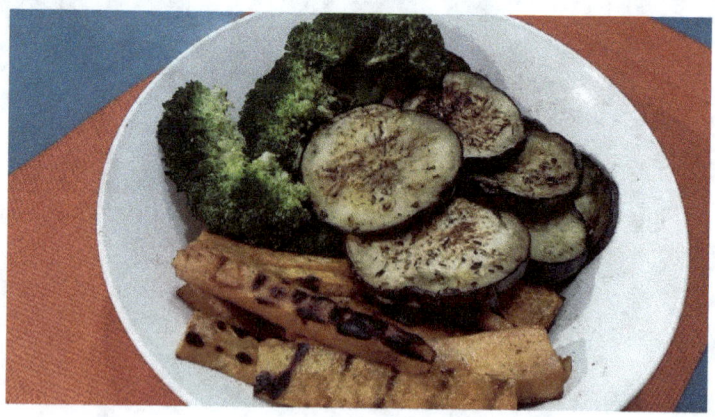

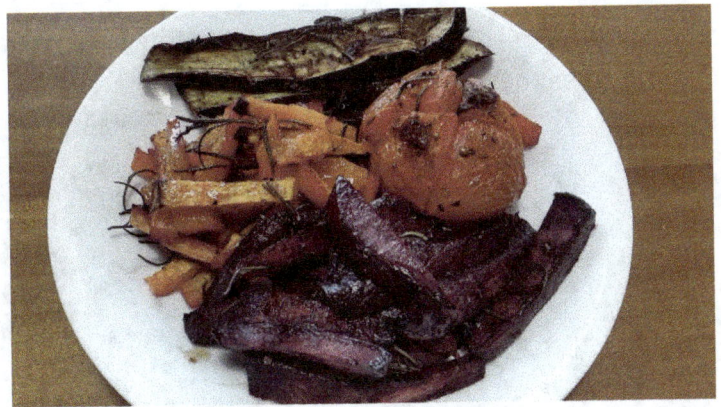

- Seasonal vegetables
- Appropriate European herbs and spices (e.g., Italian herb mix, fresh rosemary, cumin, or garam masala)
- Olive oil
- Salt and cracked pepper
- Baking paper
- Shallow oven trays
- Plastic containers for storage in fridge

Method

- Pre-heat your oven to around 180C (fan forced)
- Wash your vegetables and allow to drain
- Cover your oven tray/s with a sheet of baking paper
- Peel skins off the root vegetables
- Think about the best way to cut each type of vegetable, to ensure everything cooks in the same amount of time. For example, root vegetables like carrots and beetroot do well if cut into julienne strips like hot chips; Brussels sprouts are extra tasty if cut in half lengthways; Eggplant holds its shape if cut into circles, half-moons or long flat strips; Capsicum is good in strips too; Tomatoes are best left whole with a slit across the top.

Cauliflower should be broken up into very small florets because they take a while to cook.

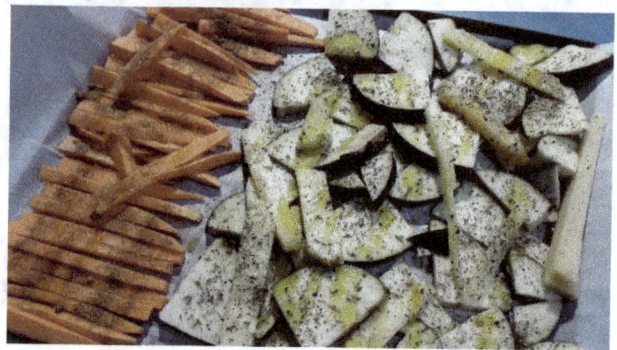

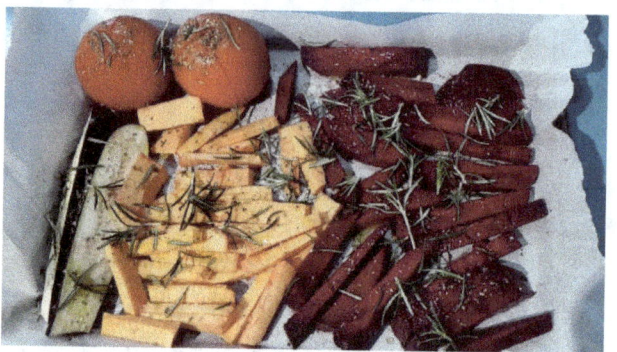

- Lay cut vegetables neatly across the baking paper in a single layer. You want every piece to get a blast of heat from the oven.
- Drizzle a little olive oil over all the vegetables. Don't cover them in oil or they'll end up an oily mush instead of crispy heaven.
- Sprinkle with herbs or spices that match each vegetable. For example, fresh rosemary goes well with beetroot and eggplant. Dried mix of Italian herbs go equally well on eggplant, Brussels sprouts, capsicum and tomatoes. Cumin and garam masala introduce a middle eastern vibe to carrots and cauliflower. Use your imagination.
- Season everything with salt and cracked pepper

- Cook for about 20 minutes, then take a look. They must be just soft enough to be poked easily with a dinner fork, and the best flavour comes when tinged a toasty brown.

- Once cooked, remove from oven and serve as a side dish, or hot snack.
- Allow leftovers to cool on the bench, then pack into plastic storage containers lined with a small piece of baking paper.
- Refrigerate until needed. Should keep for at least a week under refrigeration.

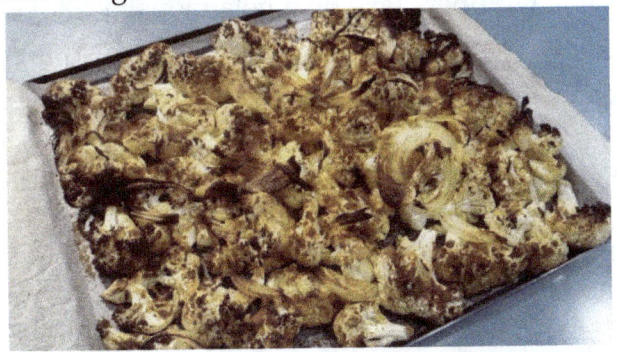

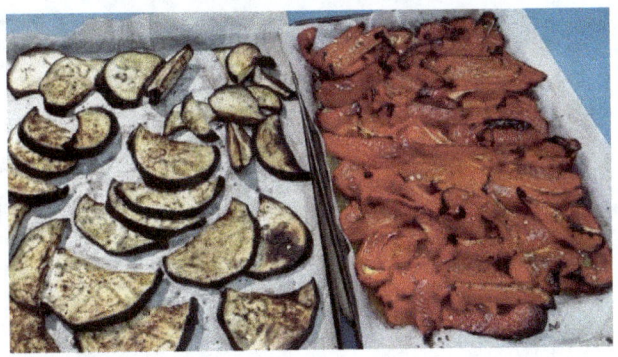

RICE NOODLE DISHES

Rice noodles are a welcome change from rice paper rolls, especially in the winter months or when you're wanting a hot plate of food. But don't have them every day if you want to lose weight.

The rice papers are there for a reason. They help restrict your portion sizes to within appropriate limits, and the unique combination of tapioca and rice flours have a special effect. When the dry rice papers are reconstituted in a water bath, the soft pliable wrappers take on a gelatinous feel, and when you eat them, your gut registers a pleasant sense of fullness. Don't underestimate the importance of these humble rice papers.

But if you start freewheeling with salads and noodle bowls, you can become very heavy handed and extra calories quickly creep into your diet. It is very easy to misjudge quantities, especially noodles, so you need to be very careful if you want to enjoy these delicious variations and continue to lose weight.

So, what does a single serving of noodles look like?

- First, let's look at rice papers. According to the pack of 10 rice paper sheets, a single serving is 2 rice papers (30g, 429kj). That's about 100 calories a serve. But in the HUNGER HERO DIET, we use 3 rice papers for every meal, which equates to 150 calories a serve (plus the filling).
- **Therefore, to replace the rice papers with rice noodles, the correct portion size must not exceed 150 calories.** This is where you need to be careful. But don't worry.

You only have to do this calculation ONCE when you start using something new, to determine what a single serve should look like.

For example, my 500g pack of rice vermicelli noodles contains 10 small bundles of dried noodles, each one weighing 50g, with 191 calories each. That's what it says on the packet. But that's an extra 40 calories I don't need, so what do I do?

Rather than muck about weighing them, I take a pair of large kitchen scissors and snip every little bundle in half. Now I have 20 serves of noodles, instead of 10, and each one is only 100 calories.

Yes! That's how it's done. When making substitutes, always err on the side of caution. And be prepared.

The same goes for the packs of flat rice noodles too. As they come in bulk packets, you will need to weigh them to get proper portions.

Whether you buy vermicelli or flat noodles, the principles are the same. But from person experience, I strongly recommend that you **divide all your noodles up into single serves as soon as you bring them home from the supermarket**. If you leave it until later, you won't bother, and you will eat too much. Yes, you will. Don't let a bowl of noodles undo all your good work.

- Read the label and work out what a single serve should be,
- Snip the dry noodles into single serves (as described), or weigh them into sandwich bags, whatever works best for you. But you MUST do this when you bring them home. If you wait until you're hungry and start cooking,

you won't be bothered. I keep mine in a large plastic storage container, so I always have them ready to use.

Okay, now you know what a portion of dry noodles looks like. But what about the other ingredients? Without the rice papers as your guide, how do you know how much to use? You could easily fill a plate or bowl with too much food, without realising it.

So, here's the trick for effective PORTION CONTROL.

- **Lay out all your ingredients** on a plate or chopping board, just as if you were about to make rice paper rolls again. Then simply use these to construct your substitute dish. You will be eating much the same food as before, but it will look and taste different because you are using those ingredients in a different way.

How to reconstitute thin vermicelli rice noodles

- place a single serve of dried noodles into a bowl
- pour over enough boiling water to cover
- to keep the heat inside, place a lid or a plate over the bowl
- leave the covered bowl to sit there and do its thing, while you prepare the rest of the meal
- after a few minutes, take a look, and give them a little stir. They should be plump and soft.
- Drain reconstituted noodles into a colander and place to one side until needed.
- Finish preparing your noodle dish.

HINT: If planning to make a soup, don't drain the noodles. Stir in a teaspoon of stock powder (or miso), then add a handful of chopped leafy greens, and a few thin slices of a favourite protein. Cover the bowl again for a few minutes to allow the extras to cook, but you can zap in the microwave for a couple of minutes if you want it piping hot. Season to taste.

How to reconstitute flat ribbon rice noodles

These noodles are thicker than vermicelli, so they need to be cooked on the stove for a few minutes.

- Pour a few cups of water into a saucepan, place on the stove, and bring to the boil
- place a single serve of dried flat noodles into the saucepan (making sure there's enough hot water to cover the noodles)
- leave the saucepan uncovered, and allow it to do its thing, while you prepare the rest of the meal
- after a few minutes, take a look, and give them a little stir. They should be plump and soft.
- Remove saucepan from heat.
- Drain reconstituted noodles into a colander and place to one side until needed.
- Finish preparing your noodle dish.

HINT: If planning to make a soup, leave the saucepan on the stove and don't drain the noodles. Stir in a teaspoon of stock powder (or miso), then add a handful of chopped leafy greens, and a few thin slices of a favourite protein. Cover and simmer for a couple of minutes. Remove from heat. Pour everything into a soup bowl. Season to taste.

Dry bowl, wet bowl, or soup broth

Asian-style noodle dishes can be 'dry' or 'wet'.
- Our version of the 'dry bowl' is a noodle salad, with a combination of warm and room-temperature ingredients.
- The 'wet bowl' contains cooked ingredients and the cooking juices, as the name suggests.
- Our noodle soups are made with a hot broth/stock into which you add noodles, Asian greens, and thinly sliced raw fish (which cooks in the hot broth and adds extra flavour).

Use any rice noodles you like, but thin vermicelli rice noodles are quick and easy. Just place in a bowl with boiling water for a few minutes. When soft, drain and put to one side. Perfect when making a wet or dry bowl dish.

When making a noodle soup, you can cheat by dropping the dry noodles directly into the hot stock on the stove. This is especially useful if using the thick rice noodles which need extra cooking time.

You can take hours making a hot broth or stock from scratch, but for our purposes, I recommend taking a short cut. The supermarket has lots of alternatives. You can buy tetra packs of liquid stock, tins of powdered stock, or the old-style stock cubes. Personally, I like the tins of vegetable-flavoured powdered stock. You only ever need a couple of teaspoons, so it's very cheap, and the flavour is mild.

Recipe: The Traveller , TUNA noodle salad

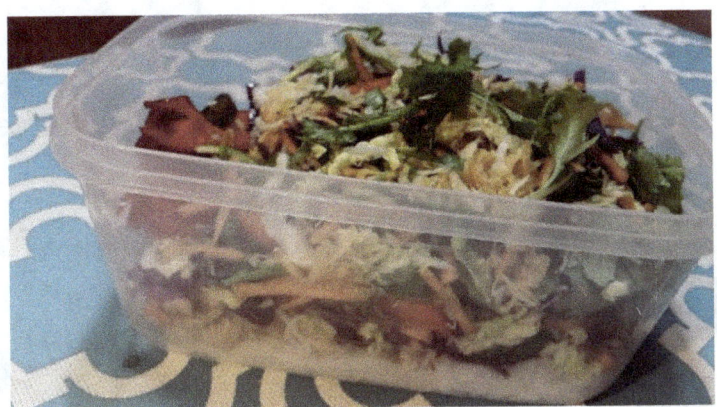

The Traveller: the perfect lunch on the go – a cold 'dry bowl' salad of TINNED TUNA with cold vermicelli rice noodles, salad, Asian dressing. Use the same ingredients you would use to fill your lunchtime rice paper rolls, but instead of rice papers, prepare a single serve of vermicelli rice noodles. Instead of yoghurt, you might like to use a liquid Asian-style salad dressing.

Method
- Line a plastic lunch box with one serving of cold, cooked vermicelli RICE NOODLES,
- top with 200g tinned tuna,
- add all the usual salad veges,
- finish with a squeeze of lemon and a drizzle of Asian-style dressing, and don't forget to pack your chopsticks.

Recipe: TUNA steak & tomato noodle salad

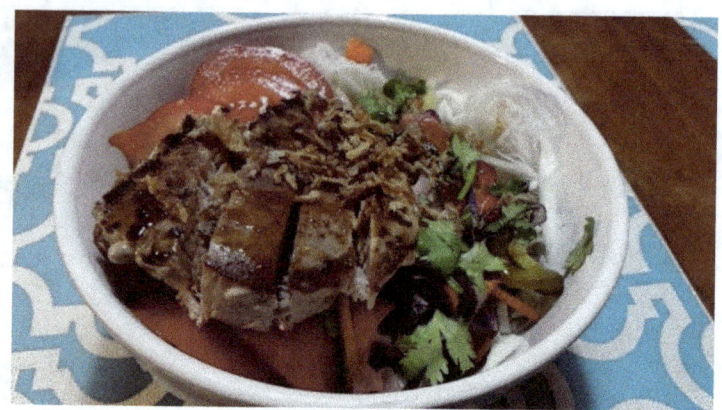

- warm pan-seared TUNA STEAK, sliced
- one serving of vermicelli noodles, drained and chilled
- cold tomato salad
- fresh herbs
- Asian dressing

Method

- Layer bowl with noodles, salad, and sliced tuna steak. Top wish fresh herbs and Asian dressing.

OPTIONAL:

- Cottage cheese
- grilled asparagus
- For a spicy hit, add a touch of chili or a few slices of pickled jalapenos.
- a sprinkling of dried fried Asian shallots.
- Can be served with warm noodles
- (Can use same recipe with pan-fried PORK SCOTCH FILLET instead of TUNA, but only twice a month.)

Recipe: TUNA steak & veg noodle bowl

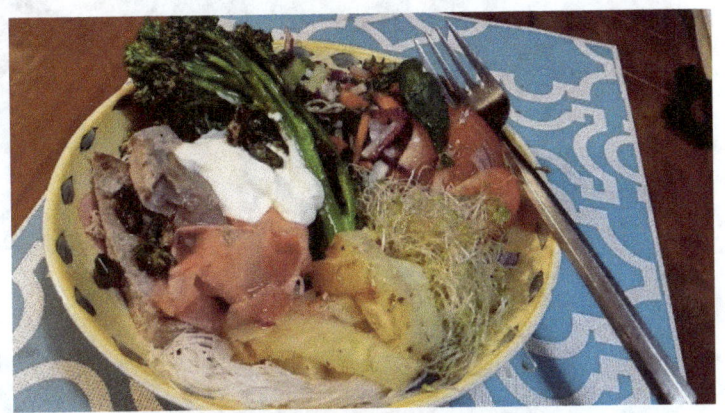

- warm pan-seared TUNA STEAK, sliced
- warm vermicelli noodles, drained
- warm sauteed broccoli and pineapple
- cold tomato salad (optional sprouts)
- pickled sushi ginger
- fresh herbs
- Asian dressing
- dollop of natural Greek-style yoghurt

Method

- Layer bowl with warm noodles, sliced tuna steak, grilled vegetables, and salad.
- Top wish fresh herbs, Asian dressing, and a dollop of Greek yoghurt.

VARIATIONS :

- Fresh lemon or lime juice instead of Asian dressing
- Add ¼ avocado and a few slices of pickled jalapenos

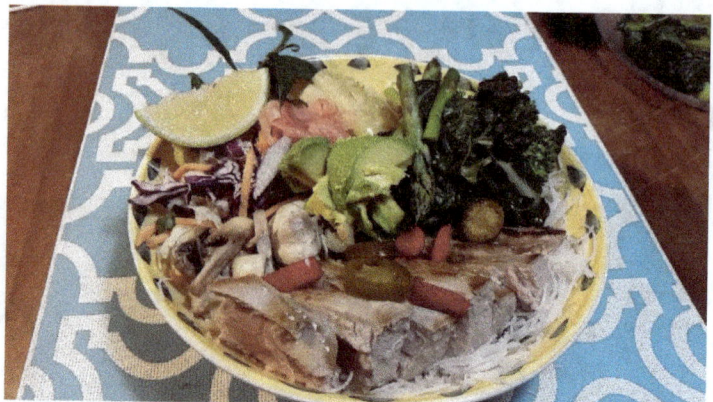

Figure 39: Tuna steak noodle bowl, avocado, pineapple, jalapenos

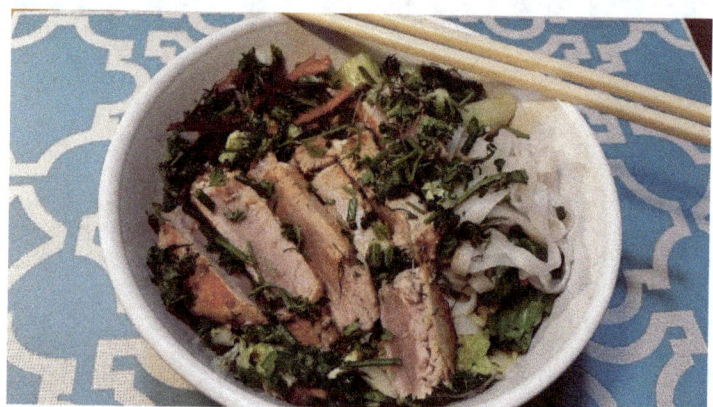

Figure 40: Pan seared tuna steak with flat noodles & veg

Recipe: PORK & avocado salad noodle bowl

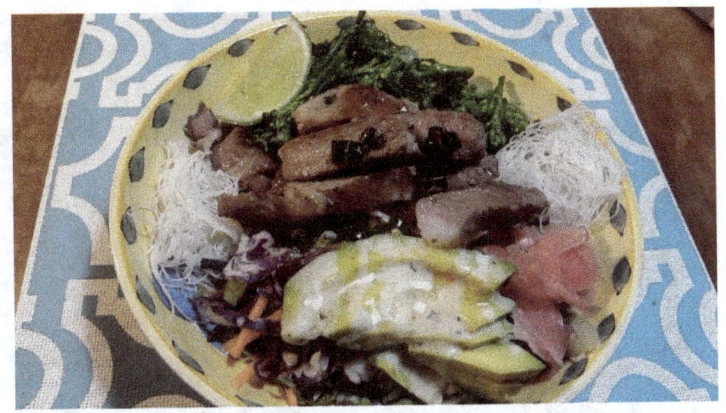

- Warm pan-fried PORK SCOTCH FILLET, sliced
- Warm sauteed broccolini
- Warm vermicelli noodles, drained
- mixed coleslaw salad, dry
- pickled sushi ginger
- ¼ sliced avocado
- Asian salad dressing
- Lime/lemon wedge
- Salt and cracked pepper

Recipe: PRAWN & braised veg noodle bowl

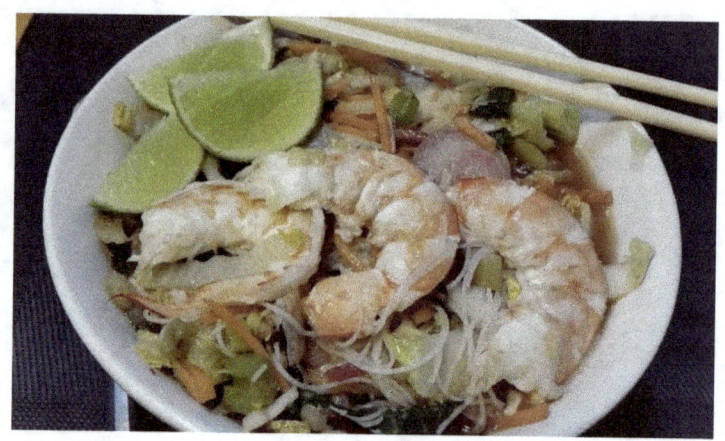

- Mixed vegetables braised in stock, in a shallow pan
- warm vermicelli noodles, reconstituted
- cooked peeled prawns, deveined
- a dash of light soy sauce
- lime juice
- a dash of fish sauce (optional)

Method

- Place braised vegetables and the pan juices into a bowl.
- Add warm vermicelli noodles and prawns.
- Add soy sauce and lime juice to taste. Fish sauce optional.

Recipe: PRAWN & Asian greens noodle broth

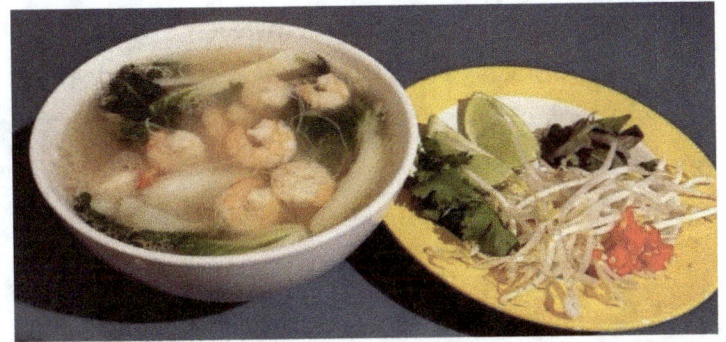

- 2 cups of boiling hot stock or broth (vegetable flavour)
- One medium saucepan
- One serve of dried vermicelli noodles
- Baby bok choy or other Asian greens
- 6 large, cooked prawns, peeled and deveined
- Light soy sauce
- Fish sauce
- Bean sprouts
- Fresh coriander and Vietnamese mint
- Lime wedges
- Teaspoon chopped fresh chili

Method

- Add vermicelli RICE NOODLES to a saucepan of boiling hot broth or stock.
- Add chopped Asian greens, and leave to cook for a couple of minutes
- Add prawns and allow to heat through.
- Remove from heat and transfer to a bowl.

- Serve with Vietnamese-style toppings (bean sprouts, coriander, Vietnamese mint, lime juice, chili).
- Balance flavours with a dash of soy and/or fish sauce.

OPTIONAL:
- Use flat ribbon rice noodles instead of thin vermicelli
- Use thin slices of raw tuna steak instead of prawns. They will cook quickly in the hot broth and add more flavour.
- Add a large teaspoon of Japanese MISO PASTE to the hot broth to create a richer flavour.

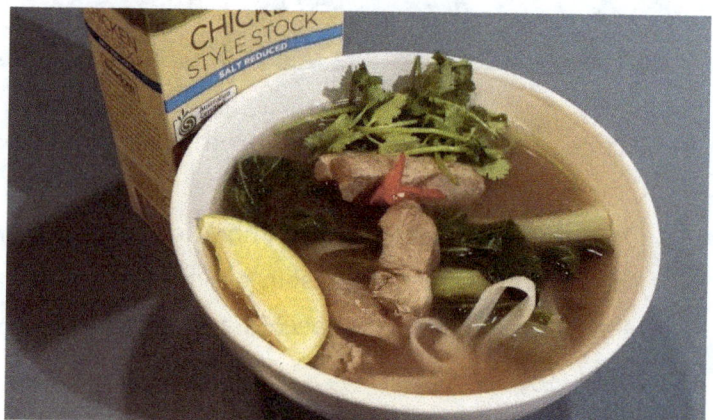

Figure 41: Asian miso broth with tuna steak and noodles

EVENING SNACKS

The afternoon and evening snacks can be swapped around. I sometimes like the simple yoghurt dip with crackers in the afternoon, but my favourite for after dinner is fruit and yoghurt.

- Almost any fruit, with a dollop of plain Greek yoghurt
- Flavours of Black Forrest Cake? Morello cherries, yoghurt, with a teaspoon of Avalanche sugar-free chocolate powder on top. **HINT**: Morello cherries are supposed to be pitted, but I usually find one small pit in every jar, so watch out.
- Rolled oats are prebiotic, incredibly cheap, and versatile as a dessert. Sprinkle raw over Greek yoghurt and fruit in summer, or as a warming porridge topped with fruit and Greek yoghurt in cooler months.
- Wanting ice-cream? Make a HALF SERVE of a protein powder diet shake. Blend the powder with ice cubes and soy milk to create a thick creamy slushy smoothie, and eat with a spoon.
- The gelatine in jelly helps to give our belly a full feeling, and these small tubs of fruit set in jelly are an excellent low-calorie snack. There are so many to choose from, such as Woolworths Two Fruits in Tropical Jelly, only 88cals per small tub. Add a dollop of creamy yoghurt to make it special.
- If your mouth wants something savoury, take ½ cup Greek yoghurt, drizzle with sweet chili sauce, and serve with a row of rice crackers. Or make a quick and easy AVOCADO DIP (see recipe).

- Another handy snack are small individually wrapped packs of cheese and crackers (bought as a box of 10 off the shelf) make for a perfect crunchy savoury snack after dinner. However, the crackers in some brands are too soft and lack the textural crunchiness, so go for the supermarket brand in our shopping list.
- In winter, a simple cup of soup might be the perfect evening snack. No doubt you have your favourites, but if you're looking for something a bit different, try miso soup. Hikari Miso Instant Miso Soup with tiny bits of wakame seaweed is an authentic Japanese miso soup. The sachets come in packs of 12 for on-the-go convenience, and all you need is hot water. Can also be used in the Asian noodle soup recipes to add an extra depth of flavour.

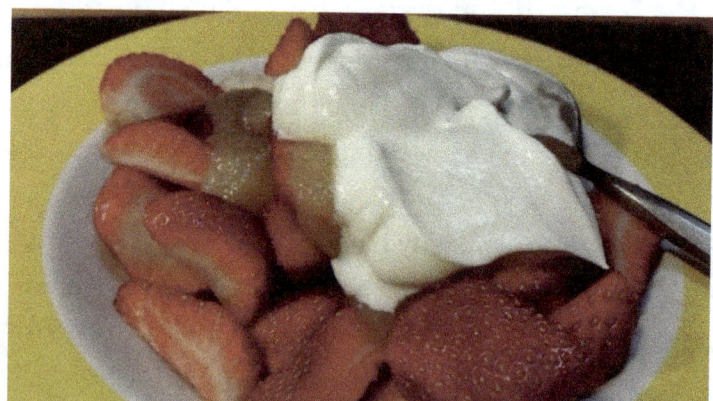

Figure 42: Fresh summer strawberries, apple sauce, yoghurt

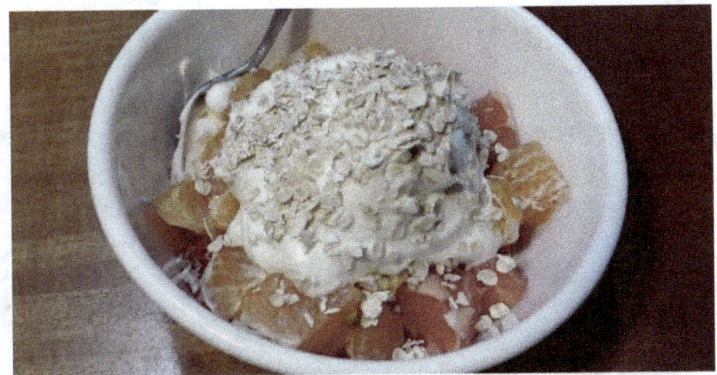
Figure 43: Diced citrus fruit, yoghurt, raw oats

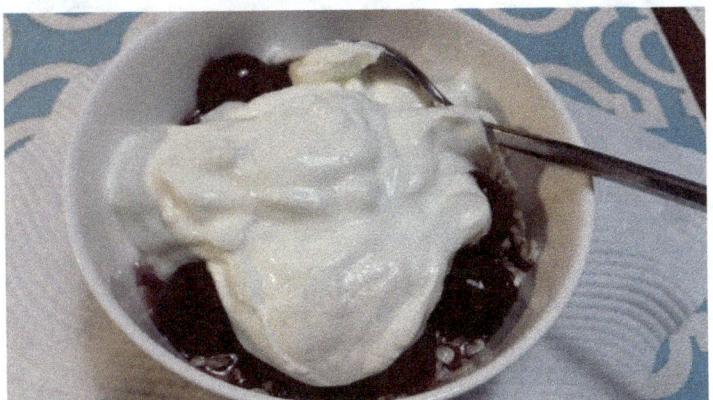
Figure 44: Hot oat porridge, Morello cherries, yoghurt

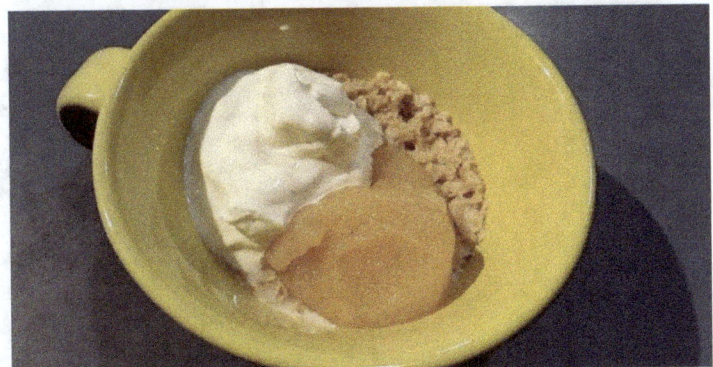
Figure 45: Hot oat porridge, apple sauce, yoghurt

Recipe: Easy AVOCADO dip

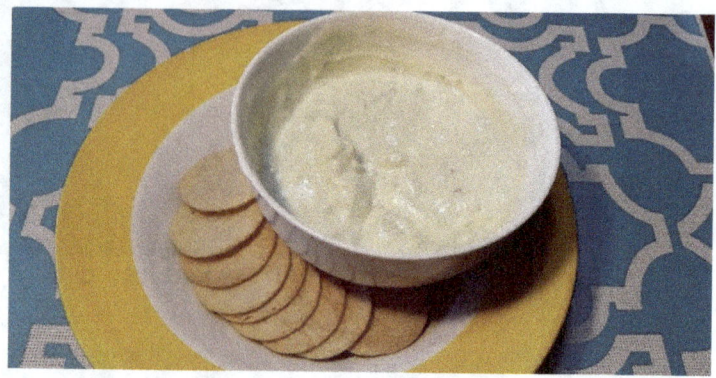

- Small bowl and whisk for mixing
- ¼ of a ripe avocado
- Half a cup of natural Greek yoghurt
- Salt and cracked pepper (chili is optional)
- One row of rice crackers (about 10)

Method

- Mix avocado with natural yoghurt, season to taste
- Serve with a row of RICE CRACKERS

VARIATION

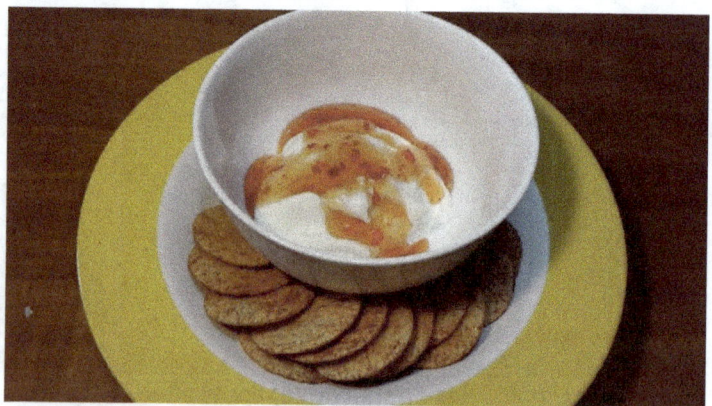

Figure 46: Natural Greek yoghurt with sweet chili sauce

Chapter 16: Let's go shopping

All items were readily available in Australia (in store and online) when this book was first published, so I hope you can find similar products wherever you live.

I've tried many brands, and bought products from all the major supermarkets in Australia, but I have to confess I keep coming back to Woolworths. Their larger stores carried all the items I needed, and surprisingly, I usually preferred their 'home brand' products for flavour, quality, and price.

I have no arrangement or connection with any company, but I have to mention this supermarket by name so you know where to find all the products on the shopping list. The other supermarket chains did not stock the core ingredients necessary for this diet, so it was easier to stick to one place for all the shopping. It just made more sense.

Of course, I am not forcing you to buy the brands that I've listed. But I tried and tested so many products, and these were my favourites. But to save you having to make a huge shop before you can start the diet, I've split the shopping list into three sections.

- CORE INGREDIENTS – you need to buy these foods before you begin the diet plan
- HIGHLY RECOMMENDED – these foods are not essential when you first start the diet, but they add variety.

But before you start bringing food home, make sure you have these in your kitchen:

- a foolscap-sized lined exercise book (as your Diet Diary),
- a pen (to write in your Diet Diary),
- a can opener,
- a small non-stick frypan,
- a chopping board,
- a good kitchen knife,
- digital kitchen scales with a flat surface (to measure food),
- a glass jar for storing tea bags,
- a few plastic storage containers of various sizes for storing leftovers in the fridge (such as tinned fish and salad vegetables),
- zip lock plastic sandwich bags for storing portions in the freezer (such as prawns and steak).

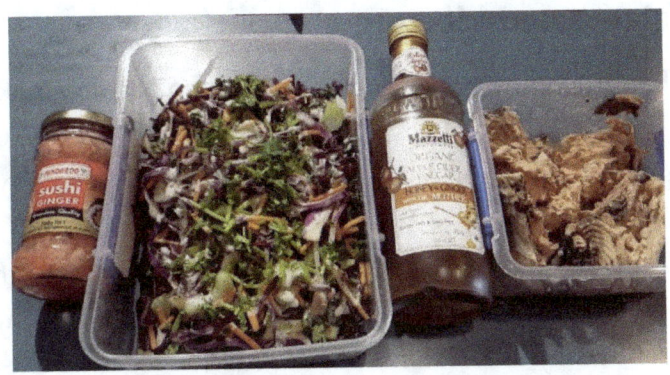

CORE INGREDIENTS

Apple cider vinegar

- Mazzetti's Apple Cider Vinegar, with the Mother, naturally fermented, or
- Woolworths Macro Wholefoods Market, certified organic, Apple Cider Vinegar, with the Mother.

Any brand will do, but I find these the most pleasant tasting. No need to buy an expensive brand from a specialty health food shop, as the supermarket brands are just as good. The 'mother' is a residual sediment formed during natural fermentation, and may contain a 'beneficial probiotic bacteria'.

Condiments, pickles, and table sauces

- Pandaroo Japanese sweet pickled pink sushi ginger, 200g jar
- Black pepper grinder
- Conimex sambal oelek hot chilli paste
- Chang's Crispy Noodle Salad Dressing, 280ml (you can taste the hint of sesame oil and soy sauce)
- Poonsin Vietnamese dipping sauce for spring rolls, 300ml (goes well with prawn salads and seafood noodle dishes)

Coleslaw salad kits, pre-cut, packaged

Buy one or more coleslaw salad kits so you can make rice paper rolls each day. These packs typically contain shredded cabbage (red, green, or Asian wombok) with carrot, celery, and a little onion.

All supermarkets carry something similar, but I've found Woolworth's stock more variety. The range changes from time to time, but they all contain a similar mix of veges. Choose one of these, or mix 2 together, e.g., the crunchy noodle coleslaw mixes well with the kaleslaw kit.

- Woolworth's Crunchy Noodle Coleslaw Kit, or
- Woolworth's Slaw Kits, Creamy Classic Coleslaw Kit, or
- Woolworth's Classic Coleslaw, or
- Woolworth's Fine Cut Coleslaw, or
- Woolworth's Four Seasons Coleslaw, or
- Woolworth's Slaw Kits Kaleslaw, or
- Woolworth's Asian Style Salad Kit, or
- Woolworth's Thai Salad Kit.

My current favourite is the Asian style salad with mizuna lettuce and wombok, the Asian version of European cabbage. But I recommend you start with the Crunchy Noodle Coleslaw Kit, as it contains a good mix of shredded cabbage, carrot, celery, onion – an ideal combination to help you lose weight. Add a bag of baby lettuce to introduce further textural variety.

DO NOT EAT THE EXTRAS: Most of these packs contain sachets of crunchy fried noodles and a salad dressing, but you won't be eating these. They contain too many empty calories. It's best if you throw them away, or just keep a few of the salad sachets in the fridge for an occasional treat. **Avoid** the Greek and Caesar salad packs, as they contain lots of calories and very little nutrition. If you want to lose weight, stick to the rules.

HINT: Once you open the salad packs, transfer the DRY salads into a large plastic container with a lid. Check the 'use-by' dates. Don't mix food with different dates in the same plastic container. And when the leftover salad starts to look a bit sad, use it in your cooking. The chopped veges are an excellent base for stir-fries and other cooked dishes, and I even throw in some leftover lettuce leaves on top. They help to steam the food underneath, while wilting down to resemble Asian greens. If you're clever, you will never throw food away again. Nothing goes to waste.

Cottage cheese, creamed

Any brand of creamed cottage cheese will do, but if unavailable, you can use ricotta for your rice cakes, but DO NOT use creamed cheese.

Fish, tinned

- Woolworths Yellowfin Tuna in Springwater, 425g.

Any brand will do, but this is my favourite. I've tried other varieties of tinned tuna across the major supermarkets, at this economical price point, and I keep coming back to the Woolworth's home brand – for texture, smell, flavour, and value for money.

Tinned tuna will be your daily staple, but avoid the small tins of tuna as they tend to be mushy. The big chunks in the larger 425g tins add extra texture to the eating experience. But you will only need about 150g per meal, so store leftovers in a sealed plastic container in the fridge (and use within 48 hours).

NB: The 185g tins are too large for one meal, and not enough for too, but they are an excellent substitute if stocks of the more popular 425g tins run low.

Only buy tuna in 'springwater', not the ones packed in brine or oil. You don't need the extra chemicals or calories, so leave them on the supermarket shelf for now. For now, avoid the small tins of flavoured tuna as they have way too many additives and calories.

Tinned salmon is an alternative to tinned tuna, but salmon is an oilier fish with more calories, and often twice the price of tuna. Red Salmon is delicious, and expensive, but if you want the occasional treat, buy the brand labelled 'wild-caught Alaskan salmon'.

I don't like the taste or texture of Pink Salmon in rice paper rolls, and the quality varies widely across brands and price points, but your cat might disagree.

Fish, frozen, tuna steaks

- Ocean Chef Yellowfin Tuna Steaks (10 wrapped portions) 1kg pack

These packs of 10 individually wrapped portions of frozen fish are an absolute must. You will wonder how you lived without them. They are so incredibly convenient.

Take a single portion out of the freezer and put it in the fridge to thaw during the day, or just leave it out on the kitchen sink for an hour before you need it. (Always sit it on a small plate as it thaws, to capture any moisture.)

When thawed, pan fry for a couple of minutes either side in a non-stick pan with some chopped up veg and you're done. A little cracked pepper, drizzle of olive oil, and there's dinner. Too easy! You don't have to be a good cook to eat well. Cook it medium or well done; it's very forgiving. I wish somebody had introduced these to me years ago when I was struggling to cook fish fillets in a pan without making a complete mess of it. (see recipe for PAN-SEARED TUNA STEAK)

Fruit

- Woolworth's Pitted Morella Cherries, or
- Marco Polo Morello Pitted Cherries.

These sour black cherries are Hunger Heroes, and a desert staple. Any brand will do. Morello cherries (bottled in juice) are widely available in most supermarkets, and even in some fruit shops. DO NOT buy tinned cherries in sugar syrup.

Aim for one or two servings of fruit every day, as your body cannot store water-soluble vitamins.

In addition to the cherries, buy a few pieces of seasonal FRESH fruit – especially those with vitamin C. Start with single-serve fruits such as kiwi fruit, oranges, mandarins, grapefruit, or stone fruit, as these are best for portion control at the start of your diet.

Pawpaw, red papaya, or pineapple are delicious and nutritious too, but if buying these larger fruit, be sure to practice proper portion control and store the leftover fruit in plastic tubs in the fridge. In the early stages of the diet, avoid bananas and apples.

Olive oil, extra virgin

- Woolworth's Australian extra virgin olive oil, 500ml, cold pressed

Any brand will do, but I prefer Italian or Australian olive oils, as heavy Spanish oils can overpower the flavour of the food. If you like the more expensive brands, grab a bargain when they go on special.

Prawns in the shell, large or medium (cooked)

Buy quality Australian wild-caught or farmed prawns IN THEIR SHELLS.

Peeling prawns is not a particularly pleasant task, but please DO NOT buy peeled prawns.

Imported peeled prawns are produced under different conditions, they lack flavour, and are often chemically treated to make them last longer. Besides, the act of peeling your own prawns is an important MINDFULNESS exercise, so make the most of it.

When shelling prawns, remember to remove the digestive tract that runs down the back from head to tail, just under the skin. It will be thick, black and grainy in wild-caught prawns, because they are free range and feeding up until they're caught; whereas the tract on farmed prawns is often only a thin white thread because they're not fed in the days leading up to their processing. For the squeamish, farmed prawns are generally a bit smaller and easier to clean than their wild-caught cousins, but wild-caught have a superior flavour.

If buying from the supermarket, they are mostly farmed prawns which have been frozen, then thawed. Do not re-freeze them, as they lose taste and texture. Thawed prawns can keep for about 2 days in the fridge once you get home, so don't buy more than 600g at a time.

If you are lucky enough to find fresh cooked wild-caught prawns that haven't been frozen, you can buy a lot more and freeze some for later use. When you get them home, divide them up into single-serve portions, seal them in plastic sandwich bags, and pop them in the freezer. Always keep prawns and other cooked food in a separate freezer compartment to raw meats, to avoid cross-contamination.

Rice cakes

- Woolworths Thin Brown Rice Cakes, Original, 150g (21 cakes, 3 cakes per serve, 86cals per serve)

Rice cakes can be THIN or THICK. The serving size is 3 thin cakes or 2 thick ones. At the start of this diet, you might find the thin ones work better for you. Visually, 3 thin rice cakes look more fulfilling than 2 thick ones, so use every trick in the book to control that hunger.

Avoid the ones made from corn or other grains. Only buy RICE cakes. Stick to the plain variety at first, but the occasional pack of flavoured rice cakes can make a nice change of pace. Any brand will do. To keep them crisp and crunchy, store in a plastic container once you open the packet. Read the labels carefully and avoid the ones made from corn or other grains.

Rice crackers

- Woolworths Original Rice Crackers, oven baked, 100g (4 rows, 1 row per serve, 104cals per serve), and
- Woolworths Multigrain Brown Rice Crackers, oven baked, 100g (4 rows, 1 row per serve, 103cals per serve)

Rice crackers, preferably plain flavour or multigrain, as these lend themselves to a variety of uses. But I like the barbeque flavour too. Always keep a couple of packets in the pantry.

These home brand products from Woolworths are my favourites, for their flavour, crispness, and price. To maintain freshness, store opened packs in a large plastic container. DO

NOT REMOVE from the trays, as this is your portion control; one row equals one portion. How easy is that?

Rice paper wrappers

- Pandaroo Vietnamese Style Rice Paper, 10 large round sheets per pack (Woolworths), or
- Valcom brand (Coles).

These dried rice paper wrappers are LARGE flat dinner-plate-sized circular sheets, sold in packs of 10 sheets. They are made in Vietnam, from tapioca, water, rice flour, and salt. They are gluten free, and one of the most important HUNGER HEROES.

We recommend 3 rice paper rolls for each meal, twice a day. That's 6 rice paper wrappers per day. There are 10 wrappers per pack, so 60 wrappers would last you 10 days. That's 6 packs. (10 days x 3 wrappers = 60 wrappers = 6 packs of 10) Buy at least 6 packs to get you started. I always buy up big when they go on special.

Woolworths and Coles keep them in the Asian food section, but if out of stock, try an Asian grocery store.

Sauerkraut, bottled

Any brand will do. Typically made in Poland, or labelled 'Polish style'. Small jars of sauerkraut are readily available in most supermarkets, whereas larger jars of Marco brand are sold in delis and fruit shops. Once you open a jar, you must refrigerate it, so choose a size to fit inside your fridge.

Many health food shops stock expensive jars of sauerkraut, but for the purposes of this diet, the supermarket brands are all you need. **TIP**: Before you buy, check the colour of the contents. If the seal is broken, the sauerkraut at the top will be a nasty brown. Don't buy it.

Tea bags, Chai spiced black

- Nature's Cuppa, Organic Chai Spiced Tea, 50 bags (Woolworths), or
- Nerada Organics, Chai Tea, 50 bags (Coles)

I've tried all the supermarket brands of chai tea and my favourite for appetite control is Nature's Cuppa, an organic spiced black tea with cinnamon, cardamon, ginger, cloves, black pepper, pure vanilla bean.

Vegetables (for cooking)

- Broccoli, silverbeet, baby bok choy, asparagus, or other greens
- AVOID onions, garlic, chives, spring onions (as they can increase appetite)

Yoghurt, Greek-style, natural full-fat

Natural Greek-style yoghurt (e.g., 1kg pot of Woolworths home brand or Farmers' Union) You can substitute with any other brand of full-fat natural Greek yoghurt, but no other type of yoghurt.

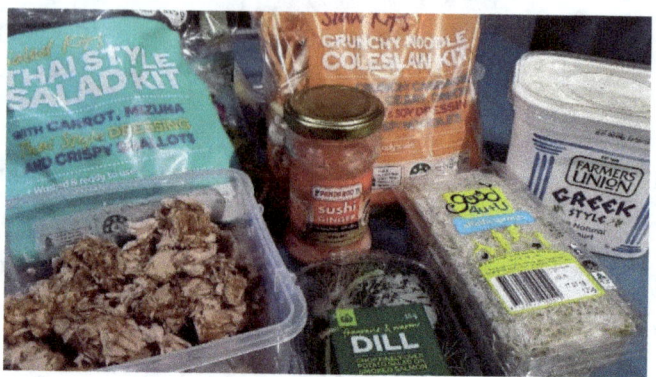

HIGHLY RECOMMENDED

Artichokes, bottled or tinned

Any brand will do. A nice low-calorie addition to recipes with a European-style flavour profile, such as a Mediterranean tomato salad.

Avocado, fresh

Avocadoes deserve a special mention. They are an inner city café phenomenon in recent years, but they need to be treated with respect. Yes, they contain lots of heart-healthy vitamins and unsaturated fats, and they can be the hero ingredient when served with seafood or a salad, but do not forget they are loaded with calories! A single portion should be ONE-QUARTER of an avocado, which is a couple of slices.

- Once you've taken your slices, pack the avo back together and cover in cling wrap, then place low down in the fridge until your next meal. It should keep for 24 hours without going brown and horrid. But if you want to be sure, keep the oxygen away from the cut flesh by sprinkling in a little lemon juice.

When buying avocadoes in a supermarket, don't expect them to be ripe. SO DON'T SQUEEZE THEM! If you do, you will bruise them and they will rot. We've all bought those ones – the ones we throw out in disgust. So don't be the avo squeezer.

Buy your avo, take it home, and leave it on the kitchen bench for at least a day, possibly two. Left out of the fridge, it will ripen. Give it a chance. With most varieties, the skin will change colour from green to brown when it's fully ripe. But I'll tell you the best way to tell if an avo is just ripe enough to eat!

- See the pointy end? See where the stalk would have attached the fruit to the tree? This is the first bit to ripen. So, VERY GENTLY, give that spot one firm press. If it doesn't give, leave it alone for another day. If it gives just a little, it's ripe enough to eat, while not being too soft. So, now you can put it in the fridge for another day or so, until you're ready to enjoy your first quarter. (You have 4 meals to look forward to.) Enjoy.

Cheese, fermented

- Woolworths Cheddar Cheese Snack, 300g, 12 pack of cheddar cheese and crackers to keep in the pantry (99calories per serve)
- Full-fat feta
- Shaved parmesan
- Low-fat cheddar slices

Coffee substitute, caffeine-free

- Nature's Cuppa Rich Roast coffee alternative, 125g, or
- Nestle Caro Extra, Delicious Cereal Beverage, naturally caffeine free, 150g

I've only seen this product at Woolworths, and the other supermarkets don't seem to have an equivalent. Make a tasty caffeine-free cup of hot mocha, with a teaspoon of Caro, a teaspoon of Avalanche Drinking Chocolate, boiling water, and a dash of soy milk. Excellent as an after-dinner drink.

Condiments, pickles, and table sauces

- A jar of sliced pickled jalapenos
- ABC Kecap Manis sweet soy sauce, 275ml.
- Light soy sauce
- Fish sauce

Cooking sauces

When making soups, broths, and 'wet' bowl dishes, a splash of Asian cooking sauces such as hoisin, oyster or light soy can add a hint of flavour to your cooking. Or you can be a little more adventurous.

- Valcom Authentic Thai Pad Thai stir-fry paste

A teaspoon of Pad Thai paste will add more complex flavours, without the heat of chili.

- Valcom Authentic Thai Tom Yum paste

A teaspoon of Tom Yum paste will provide a burst of bold flavours with a strong hit of chili.

- Jeeny's Oriental Foods Tamarind Puree, 220g

A teaspoonful of Tamarind Puree will counteract any sweetness in the dish and add a touch of sour umami flavour to any stir fry or soup.

- Woolworth's Essentials Chunky Pasta Sauce, 700g

A splash of passata or pasta sauce can enhance the flavour of veges as they cook in a pan, or when making a soup broth.

Dolmades, tinned

The vine leaves can be tough in the cheaper brands, but rice-filled dolmades make an excellent snack or light lunch when travelling.

Drinking chocolate, sugar free

- Avalanche Sugar-Free Drinking Chocolate, with stevia, 200g tin

I've only seen this product at Woolworths. The other supermarkets don't appear to have an equivalent. The rich cocoa powder is delicious sprinkled on fruit and topped with Greek yoghurt. Or add a teaspoon to the coffee substitute and make a mocha-style hot beverage.

Eggs, large, free-range

You won't be needing many eggs, but free-range are better.

Fish fillets, frozen, white fish

- Ocean Chef Hoki Fillets, 1kg pack (from Woolworths)

These wild-caught Blue Grenadier, also known as Hoki, are caught in the deep waters off New Zealand. Fillets are individually wrapped in plastic, which helps to protect the fish from freezer burn. There are lots of other frozen fish fillets to choose from in the freezer cabinets, but the fillets are not individually wrapped. For this diet, avoid the fillets with skin on, as they don't suit the recipes.

Fish, smoked salmon

- Ocean Blue Smoked Salmon from Denmark, 100g (optional)

As an afternoon snack, 50g (88cals) smoked salmon is delicious sitting on top of rice cakes and cottage cheese. As a meal, 100g (176cals) smoked salmon is a delicious alternative in rice paper rolls.

HINT: Larger packs are cheaper, but only if you are willing to divide them up into portions when you get home, without snacking. Store extra portions in plastic sandwich bags and freeze until needed.

Fruit, processed

- Jar of apple sauce
- Any tinned or bottled fruit, especially peaches and pears, IN JUICE, NOT SYRUP

The gelatine in jelly helps to give our belly a full feeling, and these small tubs of fruit set in jelly are an excellent snack (at less than 100 calories per serve). There are so many to choose from, e.g.

- Woolworths Two Fruits in Tropical Jelly (peaches and pears), 4 x120g plastic tubs, 1 tub per serve, 88cals per serve, or
- Peach in mango jelly
- Peach in strawberry jelly
- Pear in raspberry jelly
- Mango in mango jelly
- Apple in pineapple jelly

Herbal tea, caffeine-free

Try any of the more common herbal infusions, such as peppermint or camomile, or something a little different. Higher Living's Cocoa Chilli is a spicy tongue-tingling infusion of cocoa, licorice, chilli, ginger, cinnamon, fennel, anise, black pepper, vanilla, cardamon, and cloves. Available from Woolworths, 30g, 15 bags.

Herbs, fresh

Dill, coriander, Vietnamese mint, Asian basil, or fennel fronds. Avoid parsley and European basil as they don't taste very nice in Asian-style recipes. Buy from the supermarket, your local green grocer, or try growing your own.

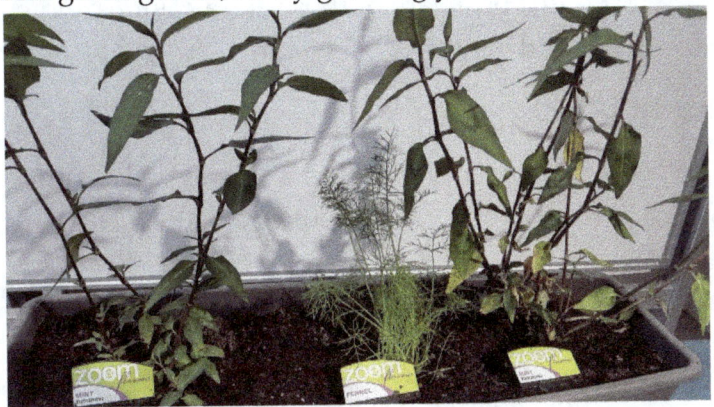

Oysters in the shell, fresh

- 6-12 oysters, fresh, if available

Don't buy them if you don't like them, and please DO NOT buy them from a supermarket. **Ask your local fish shop for fresh ones.** Season with a little cracked pepper and lemon juice. Expensive, yes, but incredibly nutritious and a source of zinc, at only 100cals per dozen.

Meat, pork scotch fillet

You won't be eating meat very often if you want to lose weight, but I always have a few single portions in the freezer for when I get the urge.

I buy small trays of pork scotch fillet steaks. Each tray is about 600g, with 4 steaks at about 150g each. With roughly 213 calories per 100g in this cut, one steak is about 320cals – more than twice the calories of your usual seafood.

When you get home, place each of the steaks into individual plastic bags (resealable sandwich-size). Lay flat to take out all the air, seal, and stack them in the freezer. You now have single portions ready to go.

Sometimes the steaks will be closer to 180g than 150g, but don't worry. Just be aware of those extra calories and cut back a little on those days.

Rice noodles

Most noodles in the supermarket are made from wheat, not rice, so be careful. Only buy rice noodles. Here are a few examples.

- Wai Wai Bihoon Rice Vermicelli, plain, pack of 10x50g bundles, 182cals, and
- Erawan Pad Thai Rice Noodles (thick ribbons)

OPTIONAL (but higher in calories):

- Wai Wai Noodles, Rice Vermicelli Instant, with crab-flavoured sachets, in a packet, 55g, 211cals, or
- Lian Pho Ga Vietnamese Style instant rice noodles, 70g, with flavour sachets, in a plastic bowl

Rolled oats or muesli, unprocessed

Any brand will do, but Woolworth's home brand is cheaper and natural.

- Woolworth's Rolled Traditional Oats, Australian
- Woolworth's Essentials Traditional Muesli, 900g

Muesli can contain lots of fruit and nuts, which are unnecessary calories when trying to lose weight. However, a small serving of UNPROCESSED muesli is a tasty and satisfying dessert porridge in winter (topped with yoghurt and Morello cherries), occasionally.

Salad vegetables, fresh

- Sprouts, mixed lettuce
- Tomatoes, cucumbers, lettuce, etc. (if making a tomato salad)

Salt, iodised

IODISED salt is fortified with iodine, an essential nutrient for thyroid health, often lacking from commercially grown vegetables. Sea salt and trendy Himalayan pink salt may taste nice, but they contain only a trace of iodine. If you use salt, choose the old-fashioned iodised salt.

Seafood, marinara mix

- Woolworth's Thawed Marinara Mix from the deli counter, 83calories per 100g

Buy 300g if stir-frying with vegetables, or reduce portion to 200g if planning to add rice noodles to the dish. Do not freeze. Refrigerate immediately, but cook it on the same day you buy it.

Soup

- Keep a few cup-a-soup varieties on hand as a quick low-calorie snack on a cold night
- Hikari Japanese Miso Instant Soup with Wakame seaweed, 12 sachets to a pack

Soy milk, regular or lite, lactose-free

Soy milk is a good lactose-free substitute for milk. Doesn't really matter if it is regular or lite, as you won't be using very much, but taste is important. Any brand will do, but my personal favourite is Sanitarium So Good.

Tofu, fried and flavoured

- Macro Honey Soy Tofu, 200g
- Macro Satay Tofu, 200g

Chilled packs of pre-cooked and flavoured tofu are versatile and low in calories. They make an ideal snack straight from the fridge, or sliced and pan fried as an alternative protein for the rice paper rolls. Any brand will do. Flavours include honey soy and satay.

Vinegar, Balsamic

Any brand will do. Ideal accompaniment for a tomato salad.

Chapter 17: Life after dieting

I developed the HUNGER HERO DIET after more than 20 years of steadily gaining weight, having struggled with post-traumatic stress disorder (PTSD), clinical depression, and debilitating arthritis.

I learnt the hard way, a long time ago, that my brain didn't function properly when I was in the grips of a full-blown depressive episode. I could act impulsively, make very poor decisions – about money, food, and people – and then suffer the consequences. So, I learnt to avoid those risky situations by staying home and keeping to myself, until the episode passed, and my cognitive functions returned to normal. The reclusiveness associated with PTSD was there for self-preservation, so going into self-imposed isolation felt natural. The solitude was a safe haven. Lonely, but safe.

I alluded to this in the INTRODUCTION; how my life had spiralled downward into a black hole so deep and dark that I was deathly afraid of never coming out. I slept my way through most of it, and lost track of time. Days morphed into weeks.

Eventually, the fog cleared, and I had survived without doing anything too drastic. But it was all a bit of a blur. I didn't remember much from all those days hidden away. After a long hot shower and a fresh change of clothes, I felt human again.

But something had changed. My clothes hung a bit loose, and the face in the mirror looked different. "OMG", I thought. "Out of a black hole comes a miracle!"

I couldn't believe it at first, but the scales confirmed it. I had lost weight. I was keen to discover how it happened, but I had no memory of the last 10 days. So, I had to become a detective and follow the trail of evidence.

I remembered shopping for food to carry me through the Xmas and New Year holidays. And I could see from the mess in the kitchen, and the overflowing rubbish bin, that I'd been feeding myself on what was in the fridge – a kilo of prawns, packs of salad, Greek yoghurt, fresh fruit, eggs, and soy milk – and frozen meals out of the freezer. I'd forgotten to buy bread, but I must have discovered how to use the Vietnamese rice papers hiding in the back of the pantry.

So, I thought, "If I lost weight so easily by eating these foods and sleeping 20 hours a day, maybe I could do it again… but without the depression and all that sleeping."

Not only did I lose weight steadily over the next few weeks, but the oh-too-regular episodes of depression became few and far between.

Surely, it couldn't be that simple? Had I inadvertently stumbled across the Holy Grail of weight loss? And could our eating habits have such a massive effect on our mental health? Yes, yes, and yes. The results were impressive, but I didn't know what made it special. So, I went in search of answers.

I read hundreds of medical research papers and developed some theories of my own. I continued experimenting on myself, adding or removing a food to see if it made any difference. Some foods triggered arthritis pain, while others worked to stifle appetite. Having read the earlier chapters, you already know it was a long and arduous road of discovery. But when I found all the answers I'd been looking for, the remaining foods made sense. They fulfilled all my nutritional needs, they satisfied all my senses, and they were a powerhouse of functional foods.

As long as I kept using the same ingredients, the depression stayed away, but if I reintroduced certain foods it came back – not as bad as before, but a much lighter version. I knew I was onto something special. In fishing terminology, I had jagged a solution to a problem plaguing millions of people, and I was compelled to share what I found. But would people follow it? Was it sustainable as a lifestyle choice?

So, what would happen if I started reintroducing some of the foods from before? What effect would that have? Could I get away with it, and still lose weight, or would the weight start coming back? Could I break the intermittent fasting rule to have coffee and a cooked breakfast at my favourite café on a Saturday morning? Could I have dinner out with friends? Could I have a few glasses of wine or a beer on a Friday night? Could I trust myself with a tub of ice-cream, or a delicious custard slice from the bakery? Can the weight loss be sustained once I reintroduce these old behaviours? The answer is YES, and NO.

After that initial 8-month weight loss phase, I tried reintroducing some old behaviours. I took it slowly, and kept it down to an absolute minimum, introducing only ONE of these off-plan behaviours ONCE a week. But even that small change was enough to cancel any weight loss that week.

"Well, that's okay," I thought. "I'll just go back and follow the diet rules next week." And yes, that did work. When I returned to the diet program, the weight loss kickstarted again. But that previous week was a kilo I didn't lose. Was it worth it? After more than 8 months of being on the diet, I have to say it was. I really enjoyed the freedom, but with freedom comes consequences.

Once I had broken the rules the first time, it became easier to do it again, and again. I could even hear my own mind debating the issue, and making perfectly valid arguments in favour of more flexible rules. But after 3 months of freedom, a couple of kilos had snuck back on, like a thief in the night.

So, what should you do? Can we have our proverbial cake and eat it too? Yes, but you need to be smart about it.

If you're happy to maintain your current weight for another week, then you can change ONE MEAL in any one week. But if you change more than that, you risk having the weight come back. Because, as sure as night turns into day, it will creep on, slowly, without you even noticing it. So, you must continue to think smart, and remain vigilant – which will be so much easier to do when you're no longer plagued by frequent bouts of depression.

Throughout the initial 8 months in the weight loss phase of the diet, I treated the entire experience as an experiment. I kept records of everything I ate. I wrote down recipes and took photos of every dish, every day. I used the same basic ingredients, but swapped them around to create something new. I kept things simple, but I did trial a stack of different dishes. You would have seen some of these in the RECIPE section, where I give a basic recipe then follow it with suggestions for variations.

Most of these variations use the same ingredients as the basic dishes, but they're combined differently, which means you can simply exchange your usual meal for one of the variations. But if you're looking to eat noodles every day, for example, the weight could start to creep back on, so be careful. Choose wisely. Eat mindfully. And enjoy your new life. Don't waste a minute of it.

Be happy!

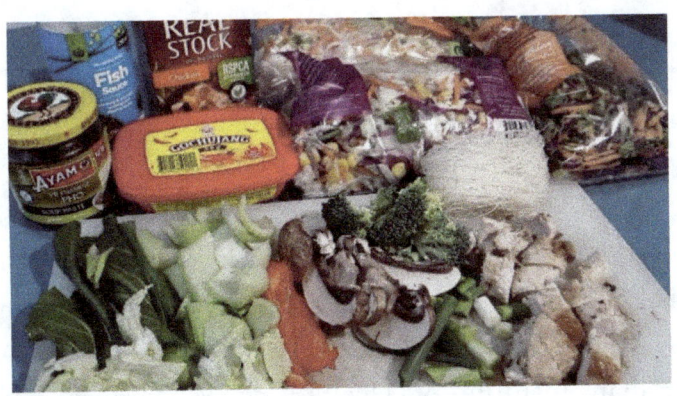

References

Abdelhamid, A. S. et al. (2018) 'Omega-3 fatty acids for the primary and secondary prevention of cardiovascular disease', Cochrane Database of Systematic Reviews. John Wiley & Sons, Ltd, (11). doi: 10.1002/14651858.CD003177.pub4.

Abete, I. et al. (2010) 'Obesity and the metabolic syndrome: Role of different dietary macronutrient distribution patterns and specific nutritional components on weight loss and maintenance', Nutrition Reviews, 68(4), pp. 214–231. doi: 10.1111/j.1753-4887.2010.00280.x.

Adcock, J. (2018) What are antioxidants? And are they truly good for us?, The Conversation. Available at: https://theconversation.com/what-are-antioxidants-and-are-they-truly-good-for-us-86062.

Afzal, S. et al. (2016) 'Change in Body Mass Index Associated With Lowest Mortality in Denmark, 1976-2013', JAMA, 315(18), pp. 1989–1996. doi: 10.1001/jama.2016.4666.

AIHW (2016) Australia's Health 2016, cat no AUS199. Australian Institute of Health and Welfare. Available at: https://www.aihw.gov.au/reports/australias-health/australias-health-2016/ (Accessed: 10 August 2019).

AIHW (2017) Weight loss surgery in Australia 2014–15: Australian hospital statistics.

Alonso, R. et al. (2008) 'Cardiovascular disease in familial hypercholesterolaemia: Influence of low-density lipoprotein receptor mutation type and classic risk factors', Atherosclerosis, 200(2), pp. 315–321. doi: 10.1016/j.atherosclerosis.2007.12.024.

American Academy of Neurology (2018) Diet shown to reduce stroke risk may also reduce risk of depression, ScienceDaily.

Available at: https://www.sciencedaily.com (Accessed: 22 April 2019).

Anton, S. D. et al. (2017) 'Effects of Popular Diets without Specific Calorie Targets on Weight Loss Outcomes: Systematic Review of Findings from Clinical Trials.', Nutrients. Multidisciplinary Digital Publishing Institute (MDPI), 9(8). doi: 10.3390/nu9080822.

Arciero, P. J. et al. (2016) 'Protein-pacing caloric-restriction enhances body composition similarly in obese men and women during weight loss and sustains efficacy during long-term weight maintenance', Nutrients, 8(8), pp. 1–19. doi: 10.3390/nu8080476.

Asano, M. et al. (2019) 'Abdominal Fat in Individuals with Overweight Reduced by Consumption of a 1975 Japanese Diet: A Randomized Controlled Trial', Obesity. John Wiley & Sons, Ltd, April. doi: 10.1002/OBY.22448.

Baliga, S., Muglikar, S. and Kale, R. (2013) 'Salivary pH: A diagnostic biomarker', Journal of Indian Society of Periodontology. Wolters Kluwer -- Medknow Publications, 17(4), pp. 461–5. doi: 10.4103/0972-124X.118317.

Bell, V. et al. (2018) 'One health, fermented foods, and gut microbiota', Foods, 7(12). doi: 10.3390/foods7120195.

Berridge, K. C. and Kringelbach, M. L. (2015) 'Pleasure systems in the brain', Neuron. NIH Public Access, 86(3), p. 646. doi: 10.1016/J.NEURON.2015.02.018.

Bliss, E. S. and Whiteside, E. (2018) 'The gut-brain axis, the human gut microbiota and their integration in the development of obesity: Review', Frontiers in Physiology, 9(900). doi: 10.3389/fphys.2018.00900.

Bostock, E. C. S., Kirkby, K. C. and Taylor, B. V. M. (2017) 'The Current Status of the Ketogenic Diet in Psychiatry', Frontiers in Psychiatry, 8, p. 43. doi: 10.3389/fpsyt.2017.00043.

Caballero, B., Finglas, P. M. and Toldra, F. (2016) Encyclopedia of food and health. Elsevier Science. Available at: https://www.sciencedirect.com/referencework/9780123849533/encyclopedia-of-food-and-health#book-info (Accessed: 13 June 2019).

Cani, P. D. (2018) 'Human gut microbiome: Hopes, threats and promises', Gut, 67(9), pp. 1716–1725. doi: 10.1136/gutjnl-2018-316723.

Carabotti, M. et al. (2015) 'The gut-brain axis: Interactions between enteric microbiota, central and enteric nervous systems', Annals of Gastroenterology. Hellenic Society of Gastroenterology, 28(2), pp. 203–209.

Chiu, S. et al. (2016) 'Comparison of the DASH (Dietary Approaches to Stop Hypertension) diet and a higher-fat DASH diet on blood pressure and lipids and lipoproteins: a randomized controlled trial1–3', The American Journal of Clinical Nutrition. Narnia, 103(2), pp. 341–347. doi: 10.3945/ajcn.115.123281.

Chousleb, E. et al. (2012) 'Reasons and operative outcomes after reversal of gastric bypass and jejunoileal bypass', Obes Surg, 22(10), pp. 1611–6.

Clarys, P. et al. (2014) 'Comparison of nutritional quality of the vegan, vegetarian, semi-vegetarian, pesco-vegetarian and omnivorous diet.', Nutrients. Multidisciplinary Digital Publishing Institute (MDPI), 6(3), pp. 1318–32. doi: 10.3390/nu6031318.

Clemons, R. (no date) 'Wheatgrass juice - food and drink | CHOICE'. Available at: https://www.choice.com.au/ (Accessed: 26 December 2021).

Crowe, T. (2018) 'Superfoods or supermyths?' Brisbane: Deakin University Alumni Seminar.

Duteil, D. et al. (2017) 'Lsd1 prevents age-programed loss of beige adipocytes', in Proceedings of the National Academy of Sciences, p. 201702641.

Ebbeling, C. B. et al. (2012) 'Effects of Dietary Composition on Energy Expenditure During Weight-Loss Maintenance', Jama, 307(24), pp. 2627–2634. doi: 10.1001/jama.2012.6607.

Epstein, L. H. et al. (2007) 'Food Reinforcement and Eating: A Multilevel Analysis', Psychological Bulletin, 133(5), pp. 884–906. doi: 10.1037/0033-2909.133.5.884.

FAO (2019) Food-based dietary guidelines, Food and Agriculture Organization of the United Nations. Available at: http://www.fao.org/nutrition/education/food-dietary-guidelines/background/en/ (Accessed: 10 May 2019).

Fenton, T. R. and Huang, T. (2016) 'Systematic review of the association between dietary acid load, alkaline water and cancer', BMJ Open. British Medical Journal Publishing Group, 6(6), p. e010438. doi: 10.1136/BMJOPEN-2015-010438.

Fildes, A. et al. (2015) 'Probability of an Obese Person Attaining Normal Body Weight: Cohort Study Using Electronic Health Records', American Journal of Public Health, 105(9), pp. e54–e59.

Flanagan, M. (2017) 'Cowpie, gruel and midnight feasts: food in popular children's literature', Irish Times.

Franks, P. W. and Atabaki-Pasdar, N. (2017) 'Causal inference in obesity research', Journal of Internal Medicine, 281(3), pp. 222–232. doi: 10.1111/joim.12577.

Franquesa, M. et al. (2019) 'Mediterranean Diet and Cardiodiabesity: A Systematic Review through Evidence-Based Answers to Key Clinical Questions', Nutrients. Multidisciplinary Digital Publishing Institute (MDPI), 11(3), p. 655. doi: 10.3390/NU11030655.

Franz, M. J. et al. (2007) 'Weight-Loss Outcomes: A Systematic Review and Meta-Analysis of Weight-Loss Clinical Trials with a Minimum 1-Year Follow-Up', Journal of the American Dietetic Association, 107(10), pp. 1755–1767. doi: 10.1016/j.jada.2007.07.017.

Frausto, D. M. et al. (2021) 'Dietary Regulation of Gut-Brain Axis in Alzheimer's Disease: Importance of Microbiota Metabolites', Frontiers in neuroscience. Front Neurosci, 15. doi: 10.3389/FNINS.2021.736814.

Gabel, K. et al. (2018) 'Effects of 8-hour time restricted feeding on body weight and metabolic disease risk factors in obese adults: A pilot study', Nutrition and Healthy Aging, 4(4), pp. 345–353. doi: 10.3233/NHA-170036.

Gardner, C. D. et al. (2018) 'Effect of Low-Fat vs Low-Carbohydrate Diet on 12-Month Weight Loss in Overweight Adults and the Association With Genotype Pattern or Insulin Secretion', JAMA, 319(7), p. 667. doi: 10.1001/jama.2018.0245.

Gearon, E. et al. (2018) 'Changes in waist circumference independent of weight: Implications for population level monitoring of obesity', Preventive Medicine, 111(June), pp. 378–383.

Hewlings, S. J. and Kalman, D. S. (2017) 'Curcumin: A Review of Its' Effects on Human Health', Foods. Multidisciplinary Digital Publishing Institute (MDPI), 6(10). doi: 10.3390/FOODS6100092.

Hill, P., Muir, J. G. and Gibson, P. R. (2017) Controversies and Recent Developments of the Low-FODMAP Diet., Gastroenterology & hepatology. Millenium Medical Publishing. Available at: http://www.ncbi.nlm.nih.gov/pubmed/28420945 (Accessed: 24 December 2019).

Howland, R. H. (2014) 'Vagus Nerve Stimulation', Current behavioral neuroscience reports. NIH Public Access, 1(2), p. 64. doi: 10.1007/S40473-014-0010-5.

Jacka, F. N. et al. (2018) 'A randomised controlled trial of dietary improvement for adults with major depression (the "SMILES" trial)', BMC Medicine. BMC Medicine, 16(1), pp. 1–13. doi: 10.1186/s12916-018-1220-6.

Japan Times (2018) Centenarians in Japan hit record 69,785 nearly 90% of them women. Available at: https://www.japantimes.co.jp/news/2018/09/14/national/centenarians-japan-hit-record-69785-nearly-90-women/#.XNTOFqQRVPY (Accessed: 10 May 2019).

Jensen, M. D. et al. (2014) '2013 AHA/ACC/TOS Guideline for the Management of Overweight and Obesity in Adults: A Report of the American College of Cardiology/American Heart Association Task Force on Practice Guidelines and The Obesity Society', Journal of the American College of Cardiology. Elsevier, 63(25), pp. 2985–3023. doi: 10.1016/J.JACC.2013.11.004.

Jiang, T. A. (2019) 'Health Benefits of Culinary Herbs and Spices', Journal of AOAC International. J AOAC Int, 102(2), pp. 395–411. doi: 10.5740/JAOACINT.18-0418.

Ju, W. (2019) 4.1: The Gut Microbiome and its Impact on the Brain - Medicine LibreTexts, Medical LibreTexts. Available at: https://med.libretexts.org/ (Accessed: 8 September 2019).

Khaw, K. T. et al. (2018) 'Randomised trial of coconut oil, olive oil or butter on blood lipids and other cardiovascular risk factors in healthy men and women', BMJ Open. BMJ Publishing Group, 8(3). doi: 10.1136/BMJOPEN-2017-020167.

Klein, A. V. and Kiat, H. (2015) 'Detox diets for toxin elimination and weight management: a critical review of the evidence', Journal of Human Nutrition and Dietetics, 28(6), pp. 675–686. doi: 10.1111/jhn.12286.

Kondo, T. et al. (2009) 'Vinegar Intake Reduces Body Weight, Body Fat Mass, and Serum Triglyceride Levels in Obese Japanese Subjects', Bioscience, Biotechnology, and Biochemistry, 73(8), pp. 1837–1843. doi: 10.1271/bbb.90231.

Kovatcheva-Datchary, P. and Arora, T. (2013) 'Nutrition, the gut microbiome and the metabolic syndrome', Best Practice and Research: Clinical Gastroenterology. Elsevier Ltd, 27(1), pp. 59–72. doi: 10.1016/j.bpg.2013.03.017.

Kristensen, N. B. et al. (2016) 'Alterations in fecal microbiota composition by probiotic supplementation in healthy adults: a systematic review of randomized controlled trials', Genome Medicine. BioMed Central, 8(1), p. 52. doi: 10.1186/s13073-016-0300-5.

Lancaster, G. I. et al. (2018) 'Evidence that TLR4 Is Not a Receptor for SaturatedFatty Acids but Mediates Lipid-Induced Inflammationby Reprogramming Macrophage Metabolism', Cell Metabolism, 27, pp. 1–15.

Le-Niculescu, H. et al. (2011) 'Convergent functional genomic studies of omega-3 fatty acids in stress reactivity, bipolar disorder and alcoholism', Translational Psychiatry, 1(4), pp. e4–e4. doi: 10.1038/tp.2011.1.

Leech, R. M. et al. (2017) 'Temporal eating patterns: associations with nutrient intakes, diet quality, and measures of adiposity', The American Journal of Clinical Nutrition. Narnia, 106(4), pp. 1121–1130. doi: 10.3945/ajcn.117.156588.

Lettieri-Barbato, D. et al. (2018) 'Time-controlled fasting prevents aging-like mitochondrial changes induced by persistent dietary fat overload in skeletal muscle', PLOS ONE. Edited by M. B. Aguila, 13(5), p. e0195912. doi: 10.1371/journal.pone.0195912.

Li, X. et al. (2016) 'Short- and Long-Term Effects of Wholegrain Oat Intake on Weight Management and Glucolipid Metabolism in Overweight Type-2 Diabetics: A Randomized Control Trial', Nutrients, 8(9), p. 549. doi: 10.3390/nu8090549.

Limbana, T., Khan, F. and Eskander, N. (2020) 'Gut Microbiome and Depression: How Microbes Affect the Way We Think', Cureus. Cureus Inc., 12(8). doi: 10.7759/CUREUS.9966.

Lo, C.-F. (2018) 'Critically Discuss the Revival of Leptin for Obesity Therapy', Psychology. Scientific Research Publishing, 09(02), pp. 217–228. doi: 10.4236/psych.2018.92014.

Lowinger, J. (2015) Why is it so hard to lose weight and keep it off?, ABC Health & Wellbeing. Available at: http://www.abc.net.au/health/ (Accessed: 3 December 2019).

Ludwig, D. S. (2016) 'Lowering the Bar on the Low-Fat Diet', JAMA. American Medical Association, 316(20), p. 2087. doi: 10.1001/jama.2016.15473.

Magkos, F. et al. (2016) 'Effects of Moderate and Subsequent Progressive Weight Loss on Metabolic Function and Adipose Tissue Biology in Humans with Obesity', Cell metabolism. Cell Metab, 23(4), pp. 591–601. doi: 10.1016/J.CMET.2016.02.005.

Mantzioris, E. and Deo, P. (2018) 'What is kombucha and how do the health claims stack up?', The Conversation, January. Available at: https://theconversation.com/

Maslow, A. H. (1943) 'A Thoeory of Human Motivation', Psychological Review, 50, pp. 370–396. Available at:

https://www.researchhistory.org/2012/06/16/maslows-hierarchy-of-needs/.

Masternak, M. M. et al. (2018) 'Dwarf Mice and Aging', Progress in Molecular Biology and Translational Science. Elsevier Inc., 155, pp. 69–83.

McNamara, R. K. (2016) 'Role of Omega-3 fatty acids in the etiology, treatment, and prevention of depression: Current status and future directions', Journal of Nutrition & Intermediary Metabolism. Elsevier, 5, pp. 96–106. doi: 10.1016/J.JNIM.2016.04.004.

McNamara, R. K. and Strawn, J. R. (2013) 'Role of Long-Chain Omega-3 Fatty Acids in Psychiatric Practice.', PharmaNutrition. NIH Public Access, 1(2), pp. 41–49. doi: 10.1016/j.phanu.2012.10.004.

Monash University (2016) Fourth Report of the Bariatric Surgery Registry v2. Melbourne, Australia. Available at: https://www.monash.edu/

Monash University (2019) Prebiotic diet - FAQs - Department of Gastroenterology. Available at: https://www.monash.edu/ Accessed: 11 September 2019).

Muhammad, H. et al. (2017) 'Dietary Intake after Weight Loss and the Risk of Weight Regain: Macronutrient Composition and Inflammatory Properties of the Diet', Nutrients. Multidisciplinary Digital Publishing Institute, 9(11), p. 1205. doi: 10.3390/nu9111205.

NHMRC (2013a) Australian Dietary Guidelines - Healthy eating for adults, Australian Dietary Guidelines.

NHMRC (2013b) Clinical Practice Guidelines for the management of overweight and obesity in adults, adolescents and children in Australia. National Health and Medical Research Council.

NIH (2019) Omega-3 Fatty Acids: Fact sheet for professionals, National Institutes of Health. Available at: https://ods.od.nih.gov/factsheets/Omega3FattyAcids-HealthProfessional/.

Paddon-Jones, D. et al. (2008) 'Protein, weight management, and satiety', The American Journal of Clinical Nutrition. Narnia, 87(5), pp. 1558S-1561S. doi: 10.1093/ajcn/87.5.1558S.

Park, C. et al. (2018) 'Probiotics for the treatment of depressive symptoms: An anti-inflammatory mechanism?', Brain, Behavior, and Immunity. Academic Press, 73, pp. 115–124. doi: 10.1016/J.BBI.2018.07.006.

Patterson, R. E. and Sears, D. D. (2017) 'Metabolic Effects of Intermittent Fasting', Annual Review of Nutrition. doi: 10.1146/annurev-nutr-071816-064634.

Pitt, C. E. (2016) 'Cutting through the Paleo hype: The evidence for the Palaeolithic diet', RACGP. The Royal Australian College of General Practitioners, 45(1). Available at: https://www.racgp.org.au/afp/2016/januaryfebruary/cutting-through-the-paleo-hype-the-evidence-for-the-palaeolithic-diet/ (Accessed: 27 April 2019).

Platell, C. et al. (2000) 'The omentum', World Journal of Gastroenterology, 6(2), pp. 169–176.

Prochaska, J. O. and Norcross, J. C. (2003) Systems of Psychotherapy - a Transtheoretical Analysis. 5th edn. Brooks/Cole.

Prochaska, J. O., Norcross, J. C. and DiClemente, C. C. (1994) Changing for Good. William Morrow and Company.

Purcell, K. et al. (2014) 'The effect of rate of weight loss on long-term weight management: a randomised controlled trial.', THE LANCET Diabetes & Endocrinology. Elsevier, 2(12), pp. 954–62. doi: 10.1016/S2213-8587(14)70200-1.

Putta, S. et al. (2018) 'Probiotics: Supplements, Food, Pharmaceutical Industry', in Therapeutic, Probiotic, and Unconventional Foods. Academic Press, pp. 15–25. doi: 10.1016/B978-0-12-814625-5.00002-9.

Rezac, S. et al. (2018) 'Fermented foods as a dietary source of live organisms', Frontiers in Microbiology, 9(AUG). doi: 10.3389/fmicb.2018.01785.

Rinninella, E. et al. (2019) 'What is the Healthy Gut Microbiota Composition? A Changing Ecosystem across Age, Environment, Diet, and Diseases.', Microorganisms. Multidisciplinary Digital Publishing Institute (MDPI), 7(1). doi: 10.3390/microorganisms7010014.

Ryan, D. H. and Yockey, S. R. (2017) 'Weight Loss and Improvement in Comorbidity: Differences at 5%, 10%, 15%, and Over', Current Obesity Reports, 6(2), pp. 187–194. doi: 10.1007/s13679-017-0262-y.

Sacks, F. M. et al. (2009) 'Comparison of Weight-Loss Diets with Different Compositions of Fat, Protein, and Carbohydrates', New England Journal of Medicine, 360(9), pp. 859–873. doi: 10.1056/NEJMoa0804748.

Salminen, P. et al. (2018) 'Effect of Laparoscopic Sleeve Gastrectomy vs Laparoscopic Roux-en-Y Gastric Bypass on Weight Loss at 5 Years Among Patients With Morbid ObesityThe SLEEVEPASS Randomized Clinical Trial', JAMA, 319(3). doi: 10.1001/jama.2017.20313.

Scheja, L. and Heeren, J. (2019) 'The endocrine function of adipose tissues in health and cardiometabolic disease', Nature Reviews Endocrinology, 15(9), pp. 507–524. doi: 10.1038/s41574-019-0230-6.

Science Daily (2018) European Association for the Study of Obesity: 'By 2035 over 4 million adults will be morbidly obese across England, Wales and Scotland', Science Daily. Available at: https://www.sciencedaily.com/

Simmons, W. K. et al. (2016) 'Depression-Related Increases and Decreases in Appetite: Dissociable Patterns of Aberrant Activity in Reward and Interoceptive Neurocircuitry', American Journal of Psychiatry, 173(4), pp. 418–428. doi: 10.1176/appi.ajp.2015.15020162.

Siscovick, D. S. et al. (2017) 'Omega-3 Polyunsaturated Fatty Acid (Fish Oil) Supplementation and the Prevention of Clinical Cardiovascular Disease', Circulation, 135(15). doi: 10.1161/CIR.0000000000000482.

Sofi, F. et al. (2018) 'Low-calorie vegetarian versus mediterranean diets for reducing body weight and improving cardiovascular risk profile', Circulation, 137(11), pp. 1103–1113. doi: 10.1161/CIRCULATIONAHA.117.030088.

Solouki, A. et al. (2018) 'One-anastomosis gastric bypass as an alternative procedure of choice in morbidly obese patients', J Res Med Sci, 23(84).

Strawbridge, H. (2013) Going gluten-free just because? Here's what you need to know, Harvard Health Publishing. Available at: https://www.health.harvard.edu/ (Accessed: 24 December 2019).

Thanarajah, S. E. et al. (2019) 'Food Intake Recruits Orosensory and Post-ingestive Dopaminergic Circuits to Affect Eating Desire in Humans.', Cell metabolism. Elsevier, 29(3), pp. 695-706.e4. doi: 10.1016/j.cmet.2018.12.006.

Thesing, C. S. et al. (2018) 'Omega-3 and omega-6 fatty acid levels in depressive and anxiety disorders', Psychoneuroendocrinology. doi: 10.1016/j.psyneuen.2017.10.005.

Thomas, D. M. et al. (2012) 'Why do individuals not lose more weight from an exercise intervention at a defined dose?

An energy balance analysis', Obes Rev, October 13(10), pp. 835–47.

Tuulari, J. J. et al. (2017) 'Feeding Releases Endogenous Opioids in Humans', The Journal of Neuroscience, 37(34), pp. 8284–8291. doi: 10.1523/JNEUROSCI.0976-17.2017.

Voelker, R. (2018) 'The Mediterranean Diet's Fight Against Frailty', JAMA. American Medical Association, 319(19), p. 1971. doi: 10.1001/jama.2018.3653.

Watson, D. L. and Tharp, R. G. (2007) Self-Directed Behavior. Belmont, CA: Wadsworth Cengage Learning.

Watson, J. (2018) Can Diet Reverse Type 2 Diabetes?, Medscape. Available at: https://www.medscape.com/

Weledji, E. P. (2016) 'Overview of gastric bypass surgery', International Journal of Surgery Open. Elsevier Ltd, 5, pp. 11–19. doi: 10.1016/j.ijso.2016.09.004.

WHO (2017) Global Health Observatory Data Repository, Prevalence of obesity among adults, BMI ≥ 30, age-standardized - Estimates by WHO region, WHO. World Health Organization. Available at: http://apps.who.int/gho/data/view.main.REGION2480A?lang=en (Accessed: 13 May 2019).

Williamson, G. (2017) 'The role of polyphenols in modern nutrition.', Nutrition bulletin. Wiley-Blackwell, 42(3), pp. 226–235. doi: 10.1111/nbu.12278.

Yashin, A. et al. (2017) 'Antioxidant Activity of Spices and Their Impact on Human Health: A Review', Antioxidants. Multidisciplinary Digital Publishing Institute (MDPI), 6(3). doi: 10.3390/ANTIOX6030070.

Zhang, J.-M. and An, J. (2007) 'Cytokines, inflammation, and pain.', International anesthesiology clinics. NIH Public Access, 45(2), pp. 27–37. doi: 10.1097/AIA.0b013e318034194e.

Zhang, N. and Yao, L. (2019) 'Anxiolytic Effect of Essential Oils and Their Constituents: A Review', Journal of Agricultural and Food Chemistry, June(13), p. acs.jafc.9b00433. doi: 10.1021/acs.jafc.9b00433.

Zhao, G. et al. (2011) 'Waist circumference, abdominal obesity, and depression among overweight and obese U.S. adults: national health and nutrition examination survey 2005-2006', BMC Psychiatry. BioMed Central Ltd, 11(1), p. 130. doi: 10.1186/1471-244X-11-130.

About the author

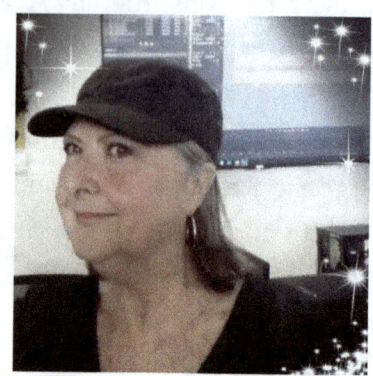

Kathryn M. James

MASR(Health), BScBiomedical(Hons), GDipA(Coun), GDipFDRP

Kathryn M. James is an award-winning author who takes a unique and colourful approach to the challenges of obesity and depression.

She survived a series of violent traumatic events during an international career in IT and resort management, and returned to Australia with debilitating health issues. Frustrated by a perceived lack of cohesion in the medical system, and unwilling to just give up, Kathryn went in search of her own answers – completing five biomedical and behavioural science degrees over the next 10 years.

This book is the culmination of that highly advanced multi-disciplinary training, which she combines with the latest medical research, her knowledge of other cultures, and her own lived experience. The HUNGER HERO DIET is a compelling read, offering hope to millions of people.

Website: https://KMJamesWriter.com/
Email: KMJamesWriter@outlook.com